Senior Fitness

SAFELY STARTING
A NEW SENIOR FITNESS PROGRAM

Suzy Campbell

Fitness With Suzy
7735 Willow Cove Circle
Las Vegas, Nevada 89129
Suzyzumba1@gmail.comm

Book Layout ©2017 BookDesignTemplates.com

Ordering Information:
Quantity sales. Special discounts are available on quantity purchases by corporations, associations, and others. For details, contact the publisher at the address above.

Senior Fitness
Safely Starting a New Senior Fitness Program—1st ed.
ISBN9798851776298 (Softcover)

The author generated this text in part with GPT, OpenAI's large-scale language-generation model. Upon generating draft language, the author reviewed, edited, and revised the language to their own liking and takes ultimate responsibility for the content of this publication.

Before beginning or adjusting any fitness program, please consult with a licensed health professional who can provide advice based on your personal medical history. This book provides general information to increase awareness, and educate readers. There are differing views on many of the topics covered in this book including benefits, and risk of injury. The publisher assumes no responsibility and expressly disclaims all warranties of any kind, whether expressed or implied to the full extent permitted under applicable laws, relating to your use of this book. Please consult with a health professional if you have any negative side effects.

To Russell, My Inspiration

Contents

OVERVIEW FOR A SENIOR'S FITNESS PROGRAM

Hey there, super seniors! Ready to kick some exercise butt and show the world that age is just a number? You bet you are!

Now, some folks might think that exercise is only for the young and spry, but let me tell you, my awesome friends, it's never too late to get moving and grooving. We're about to embark on a fitness adventure that will make you feel like a superstar!

Before we dive in, let's lay down some ground rules. Think of this as your roadmap to a healthy and active life. I've got six key elements to cover, so grab a chair (or not, we'll get to that later) and let's get started!

1. **Get the Green Light**: Before you become a fitness superstar, it's always a good idea to consult with your healthcare provider. They'll make sure you're ready to rock and roll and provide guidance based on your unique needs and any medical conditions you may have. Safety first!

2. **Warm-Ups**: Just like a car needs a warm-up before hitting the road in cold weather, your body needs a warm-up before exercise. It's like a pre - party for your muscles, joints, heart & lungs. You'll start with a 5-10 minute warm-up that gets the blood pumping & the joints moving. This can include light cardio exercises like the "Brisk walking extravaganza ", or ""Cycling or elliptical fiesta"! Also, include movements that gently mobilize your joints, such as arm circles, & hip rotations. This helps to lubricate your joints & improve range of motion. During the warm-up, gradually increase the intensity & speed of your movements, but avoid pushing yourself too hard or causing

fatigue. We're not competing in the Olympics just yet. We're not aiming for a world record - we just want to warm up those muscles & joints. So let's shake off that sleepiness, wiggle those limbs, & rev up your engines!

3. Cool Down & Flexibility: After your workout, it's time for a cool-down. We're not talking about sipping iced tea (although that sounds delightful), but rather doing light exercises and static stretches. This helps your muscles recover and prevents soreness. Plus, it gives you an excuse to strike a pose and feel like a fitness guru! Here's a few examples of stretches to get you started:

- Let's start with those "**Calves**." Find a wall or a sturdy friend to lean against. Extend one leg back, press that heel into the ground, and feel the stretch in your calf. Hold it for 20 to 30 seconds
- Now, for those "**Hamstrings**". Bend over and reach for your toes or ankles and say hello to those Hammys! No worries if you can't touch your toes. Just go as far as you can and hold that stretch like a cool statue!
- Next up, the "**Quadriceps**" – those mighty muscles at the front of your thighs. Stand up tall and bend one knee, grabbing your ankle (like a pro!) and gently pulling it towards your behind. Hold it steady for the magic 20 to 30 seconds!
- Now, let's give our "**Chest**" some love. Find a doorway, place your forearm on the frame (palm facing up), and lean in slightly. You'll feel that stretch across your chest like you're giving it a big ol' hug!
- Ah, the "**Shoulders**" and "**Back**" are up next! Clasp your hands together in front of you and reach forward as far as possible. Feel that stretch in your upper back and shoulders – it's like a fantastic stretchy hug for your upper body.

Remember, folks, these stretches are all about relaxation and feeling good. No need to rush – just take your time and enjoy the moment. Hold each stretch for those 20 to 30 seconds, and your muscles will thank you later by being all happy and cozy.

And guess what? Not only do these stretches make you feel like a flexible Gumby, but they also prevent those pesky muscle soreness monsters from sneaking up on you later. It's like your secret weapon against post-workout grumbles!

So, give yourself a pat on the back (figuratively, of course) for nailing those cool-down stretches. You've leveled up your flexibility game, and you're ready to conquer the day like the magnificent fitness star you are! High-five

4. **Low-Impact Cardiovascular Exercise**: Who says cardio is only for the youngsters? We'll focus on low-impact exercises that are easy on the joints but still get that heart pumping. Brisk walking, dancing, swimming, or cycling are all fantastic options. It's like a dance party for your heart, and you'll be rocking it!

- First up, we've got the **"Brisk Walking Bonanza"**! Take a stroll like you're late for the world's coolest party, but remember, no running allowed – we're keeping it gentle on those joints!
- Now, let's groove with some **"Dancing Delight"**! Shake your booty and move like nobody's watching – you're a dancing superstar! Whether you're a funky chicken or a smooth salsa dancer, it's all about having a blast!
- And how 'bout some **"Swimming Shenanigans"**? Jump into the pool and splash around like a playful dolphin. Swim your way to fun and fitness – it's like a mermaid adventure!
- For all you water lovers, **"Water Aerobics Extravaganza"** is the name of the game! It's like a dance party, but in the water! Jump, twist, and wiggle in the pool like a water wizard!
- Oh, we can't forget the **"Cycling Celebration"**! Hop on a bike and pedal your way to excitement. Whether it's outdoors or a stationary bike, you'll be a cycling superstar in no time!

- And if you want to feel like you're climbing a mountain but without the actual mountain, try the **"Treadmill Trek"** or the **"Elliptical Expedition"**! Go at your own pace and conquer those machines like a fitness conqueror!

The best part? These exercises are kind to your precious knees and shoulders. No stress allowed – we're all about feeling good!

Now, let's talk about the amazing benefits of these activities.

- First off, they'll boost your **"Cardiorespiratory Fitness"** – a fancy way of saying your heart and lungs will be super happy!
- And hey, if you're on a mission to **"Lose Weight,"** these exercises can be your trusty sidekick! Combine them with healthy eating, and you'll be unstoppable!
- Oh, but wait, there's more! These workouts are like a shield against the sneaky villains called **"Type 2 Diabetes," "Coronary Heart Disease," "Breast and Colon Cancer,"** and **"High Blood Pressure."** Show 'em who's boss!
- Last but not least, these exercises are like ninja moves against **"Falls."** You'll have the balance of a graceful acrobat – no banana peels can stop you!

So, how much of this awesomeness should you do each week? Aim for 150 to 300 minutes of moderate-intensity exercise or 75 minutes of vigorous exercise. You've got this!

Alright, my exercise champions, go out there and conquer the world of fitness! You're gonna rock those low-impact workouts like nobody's business! High-fives all around!

5. **Strength Training**: Time to show those muscles some love! Strength training is all about building strength, boosting your metabolism, and improving your body composition. We'll start with bodyweight exercises or light weights, targeting all major muscle groups. Think of it as a little workout for each part of your body—arms, legs, core, the whole shebang!

Hey there, fellow fitness enthusiasts! It's time to get strong and show off those muscles! Strength training is the name of the game, and boy, does it come with a ton of amazing benefits!

- First off, it's like the ultimate muscle bodyguard – **"Preserving Your Muscle"** like a fortress! Keep those muscles strong and sturdy, so you can carry all the grocery bags in one trip – no problem!
- And guess what? Strength training can do a magic trick – **"Increasing Your Metabolism"**! Yup, that means your body becomes a calorie-burning machine – like a furnace cranking up the heat!
- Now, let's talk about **"Body Composition"** – the art of having more muscle and less fat. It's like sculpting your body into a masterpiece – say hello to those strong muscles and wave goodbye to unwanted fat!
- Oh, and here's a bonus perk: **"Strengthening Your Bones"**! It's like giving your skeleton a high-five – keeping it tough and unbreakable!
- But wait, there's more! **"Reducing Your Resting Blood Pressure"** – it's like a zen garden for your heart. So, no more stressing over high blood pressure – you're as cool as a cucumber!
- And brace yourself for this one: **"Elevating Your Mood and Self-Confidence"**! Strength training gives you an extra boost of happiness and self-belief. You'll be strutting around like a rockstar, trust me!

Now, let's dive into the fun stuff – the actual exercises! Start with "Resistance Exercises" using your own body weight or some light weights. It's like lifting feathers – easy peasy!

Remember, we're not lifting trucks just yet! Do 8 to 12 repetitions of each exercise for one to two sets. When you are ready for it, try to add a third set!

You've got plenty of other options – you can use **"Resistance Bands"**, **"Dumbbells"** or give those **"Weight Machines"** with low resistance a try. It's like playing with fitness toys – woohoo!

Now, let's make sure we cover all our bases!

- Work on those **"Lower Body"** muscles – legs and butt, we're lookin' at you! Flex those glutes and strut like a proud peacock!
- Next up, we've got the **"Upper Body"** brigade – chest, back, and shoulders! Show off your strength and rock those exercises like a fitness guru!
- Don't forget those **"Arms"** – biceps and triceps, you're up! It's like showing off your muscles at the beach – hello, beach biceps!
- And last but not least, let's tighten that **"Core"** like a superhero with a six-pack!

Alright, my fierce fitness seniors, you've got the power to rock this strength training game! Just 2 to 3 non-consecutive days a week, and you'll be flexing those muscles like a champ! Let's do this!

6. **Balance and Stability**: You know what they say, "Balance is the key to a harmonious life!" We'll incorporate exercises that improve your balance and stability. It's like having your own personal acrobat training. From standing on one leg to walking heel-to-toe or trying out some yoga or Tai Chi moves, we'll have you balancing like a pro! Today, we're gonna talk about the secret sauce of life – "Balance"! No, not balancing plates on our heads (though that could be fun), but balancing our bodies like acrobats!

Picture yourself as a circus superstar, ready to conquer the tightrope! Well, not exactly a tightrope, but we'll do some exercises that'll make you feel like you're in the circus – in a good way!

- First up, it's the **"One-Leg Stand Spectacular"**! Stand on one leg like a flamingo striking a pose. Flap your arms if you want – you'll look super cool!
- Now, for some **"Heel-to-Toe Walking Wonderment"**! Pretend you're walking on a straight line like a graceful ballerina or a high-wire act. Just put one foot in front of the other – easy peasy!
- But hey, we've got some zen moves too – it's **"Yoga Time"**! Stretch and twist like a happy pretzel. Strike a pose like a warrior, or maybe even a downward dog (it's not as scary as it sounds, I promise)!
- And let's not forget about **"Tai Chi Fun"**! Move like a slow-motion ninja, flowing from one graceful stance to another. You'll feel like you're floating on air!

These exercises are like training to be a real-life acrobat – except without the circus tent and scary clowns (phew!). They'll make your balance and stability rock-solid!

Why is balance important, you ask? Well, you'll be steady as a rock and less likely to trip and stumble. No falling for us, thank you very much!

So, let's wobble, wiggle, and waltz our way to balance mastery! You'll feel like a graceful dancer or a ninja warrior in no time!

Get ready to conquer the world of balance – one step at a time! You're gonna be a balancing superstar! Woohoo!

Gradual Progression: Rome wasn't built in a day, and neither will your fitness empire. You'll start slow and gradually increase the intensity, duration, and frequency of your exercises. Remember, listen to your body, and if something feels off, take it easy. Safety first, remember?

So there you have it, my fabulous exercisers! Your guide to becoming fit and fabulous. Remember, this is all about having fun, staying healthy, and feeling amazing in your own skin. Don't worry about comparing yourself to others—this is your fitness journey!

Let's get ready to rock those sneakers and embrace the joy of exercise. Together, we'll show the world that age is just a number, and we seniors can rock the fitness world like nobody's business!

THE ABC'S OF WORKING OUT

Hey there, fitness enthusiasts! Let's dive into the ABCs of working out. No, we're not talking about the alphabet here. We're talking about Alignment, Breathing, and Control. These three amigos can seriously up your workout game while keeping you safe. So let's break it down.

First up, we have **"A" for Alignment**. Now, alignment is all about maintaining the right posture and positioning during exercises. We want to keep those joints, muscles, and connective tissues happy and strain-free. Here are some simple things to keep in mind:

1. Keep your spine in a neutral position. That means your head, neck, and back should be in a natural and straight line. No slouching, okay?
2. Engage those core muscles. Activate your abs and back muscles to provide stability and support. It's like giving your body a nice, cozy hug.
3. Brace yourself! Nope, not for impact, but to stabilize your spine. Think of it as sucking in your navel towards your spine.
4. Pay attention to your joints. Knees, hips, shoulders, you name it. Make sure they're in a stable and aligned position. No wobbly joints allowed!

Moving on to **"B" for Breathing**. Breathing is super important for getting the most out of your workout. Here's how to do it right:

1. Take deep breaths. Inhale through your nose and let your belly expand like a balloon. Then exhale through your mouth. It's like blowing out birthday candles, but without the cake.
2. Coordinate your breath with your movements. When you're lifting something heavy, like a weight, breathe out. And when you're relaxing, breathe in. It's like your breath is dancing with your workout moves. Inhale, exhale, repeat!

Last but not least, we have **"C" for Control**. This is all about staying in the driver's seat during your exercises. Buckle up and check these out:

1. Take it slow and steady. No need to rush. Perform your exercises in a controlled manner, focusing on each muscle for about 3 to 4 seconds for both directions of the movement. It's like enjoying a slo-mo action movie with your muscles as the stars.
2. Embrace the full range of motion. Move through the entire motion of each exercise, but don't compromise your form or alignment. It's like going from point A to point B without taking any shortcuts.
3. Get that mind-muscle connection going. Concentrate on the muscles you're working on and really feel them. It's like having a little chat with your muscles, telling them, "Hey, you're doing great!"

By following these ABCs in your workouts, you'll be a pro in no time. They'll improve your technique, reduce the risk of injury, and make your workout sessions even more rewarding. Just remember, different exercises may have their own special variations, so it's always good to consult a fitness pro for guidance tailored to your specific workout style.

Keep those ABCs in mind, stay active, and have fun with your workouts. You're on your way to becoming a fitness superstar!

REPS-SETS-REST

Alright, my exercise buddies, let's break down the jargon and have a little fun with "reps," "sets," and "rest." These are the secret codes of the workout world, and today, I'm decoding them just for you!

Reps

First up, we have "reps," short for repetitions. Think of reps as your exercise superheroes, showing off their moves. It's the number of times you perform a specific exercise without taking a break. In general, use a weight that you can do at least 8, and no more than 15 reps.

Sets

Now, let's talk about "sets." Sets are like squads of reps, working together to achieve greatness. They help organize your workout and keep things in check. Picture this: you decide to do 3 sets of 10 push-ups. Here's how it goes down. You do 10 push-ups, take a little breather, then repeat another 10 push-ups. Take another rest, and finally, finish strong with the last 10 push-ups. Boom! You just conquered 3 sets of push-ups like a champ!

Rest

But wait, there's more! We can't forget about "rest." Rest is like your workout's best friend. It's that sweet time when your body gets to recover and recharge. Resting between sets or exercises is super important. It helps you maintain good form, avoid getting too tired, and get ready for the next set. The length of your rest time depends on your fitness level, the intensity of your exercise, and your goals. So take a breather, catch your breath, and get ready for the next round!

Remember, the specific numbers of reps, sets, and rest periods can vary depending on what you're aiming for. If you're all about building strength, you might go for lower reps (like 6 to 8 reps per set) with heavier weights and longer rest periods. But if endurance is your game, you might opt for higher reps (around 12 to 15 reps per set) with lighter weights and shorter rest periods.

It's also important to have rest days between your strength workouts. If you experience delayed onset muscle soreness (DOMS), participate in other activities which will let your over-used muscles rest and repair (Swim, walk, dance, fitness class).

To keep things on track and make sure you're using the right parameters for your exercises, it's a good idea to follow a structured program. And hey, if you're not sure where to start, don't sweat it! That's what fitness professionals and trainers are there for. They can help you design a workout routine that fits your needs and keeps you on the right path.

So there you have it, my exercise pals! Now you're in the know about reps, sets, and rest. Use this knowledge wisely, keep pushing yourself, and remember to have fun along the way. You've got this!

PREPARATION AND RECOVERY GUIDELINES

Hey there, fitness fanatics! Let's talk about the two magic words: pre-workout **preparation** and post-workout **recovery**. Trust me, they're both very important in your fitness journey. We'll focus on hydration and nutrition because they're the cool sidekicks that make everything better. Are you ready? Let's dive in!

Pre-workout Preparation

Hydration

Hydration is key. Make sure you drink water throughout the day to stay properly hydrated before your workout. Want a secret tip? Aim to gulp down around 16 to 20 ounces (that's 500 to 600 milliliters) of water 2 to 3 hours before you exercise. Then, about 15 to 30 minutes before you start sweating, drink another 8 to 10 ounces (that's 250 to 300 milliliters) of water. It's like giving your body a big ol' drink of superhero power!

Pre-workout meal/snack

Now, let's talk about pre-workout fuel. Your body needs the right combination of carbs for energy and protein for muscle repair. So, munch on a balanced meal or snack 1 to 3 hours before you hit the gym. Think whole grains, fruits, veggies, lean proteins, and healthy fats. Avoid heavy, greasy, or fibrous meals that might make you feel like a grumpy monster during your workout. We don't want that, right?

Post-workout recovery

Hydration

Hydration, once again, takes the stage. After your workout, make sure you replenish your fluid levels by drinking water. Try to chug down at least 16 to 24 ounces (that's 500 to 750 milliliters) of water for every pound (or 0.5 kilograms) you lost during exercise. And if you went all-out with an intense or long workout, consider sipping on a sports drink with electrolytes to replenish those sodium and potassium levels.

Post-workout meal/snack.

It's time to refuel your body with a balanced meal or snack within 1 to 2 hours after your workout. This will help your muscles recover and restore your energy levels. Fill up on a combination of carbs (to restock glycogen stores) and proteins (for muscle repair).

Aim to consume 20 to 30 grams of high-quality protein. Lean meats, poultry, fish, dairy products, legumes, and plant-based options like tofu or quinoa are your protein-packed pals..

Oh, and if a full meal isn't possible right away, go for a yummy snack like a protein shake or bar, Greek yogurt, or nuts. Mmm, delicious!

Remember, everyone's body is unique, so listen to what yours is telling you. Adjust your hydration and nutrition strategies based on your individual needs. Keep an eye out for any dietary restrictions, allergies, or intolerances you might have.

And hey, hydration and nutrition aren't just for pre- and post-workout moments. They're your buddies all day long, supporting your performance and recovery.

If you need some extra guidance, consider consulting a registered dietitian or nutritionist. They can give you personalized tips based on your goals, dietary needs, and exercise routine.

HOW DO I PROGRESS?

Hey, rockstar! Three months of consistent exercise? That's amazing! But hey, let's spice things up a bit because we don't want your progress to hit a plateau. Time to add some pizzazz to your workout routine with these super fun ways to modify and progress:

1. **Amp up the intensity, baby!** Give your muscles a challenge by gradually increasing the intensity of your exercises. If you're an old pro at strength training, grab some heavier weights or resistance bands. And for cardio exercises, crank up the speed, resistance, or incline. If you've been strolling, let's upgrade to a power walk or sprinkle in some sprints. Zoom, zoom!

2. **Say hello to variety!** Spice up your routine by introducing new exercises or variations. It's like inviting new dance moves to the workout party. Target different muscles and keep things interesting. Instead of plain old squats, try fancy variations like sumo squats or Bulgarian split squats. And hey, let's not limit ourselves to one activity. Dive into swimming, cycling, or join a cool group fitness class. Variety is the spice of exercise!

3. **Ready for some numbers games?** Increase your repetitions or sets, my workout whiz! This will build your endurance and push those muscles even further. If you've been doing 10 reps of an exercise, let's level up to 12 or 15. Feeling brave? Add an extra set for each exercise. You've got this!

4. **Modify, modify, modify!** Adjust those exercise variables to shake things up. Slow down the tempo of your movements. Explore a bigger

range of motion and surprise those muscles. And hey, let's get adventurous with unstable surfaces like a wobbly stability ball or a bouncy balance pad. It's like exercising on a trampoline, but without all the jumping!

5. **Get functional**! Time to bring your workout to the real world. Include exercises that mimic everyday movements and boost your functional fitness. Squats, lunges, step-ups, or even pretending you're carrying those heavy grocery bags. It's like turning your workout into a training session for real-life activities.

6. **Need some guidance?** Seek the help of a certified personal trainer or fitness pro! They're like workout wizards who can assess your current routine and design a new one tailored just for you. They'll sprinkle in new exercises and techniques to keep you challenged and on the road to success. Plus, they'll make sure you're exercising safely and effectively.

Just remember, take it easy and listen to your body. Progress gradually and if anything feels funky or uncomfortable, make adjustments or seek professional help. I want you to be safe and feel awesome on your fitness journey.

Now, go out there and rock your modified workout routine!

BALANCE EXERCISES

Hey there, balance enthusiasts! We're about to embark on a journey of stability, coordination, and body awareness. Get ready to add some balance exercises to your routine and conquer the world (or at least your living room). Here are a few examples to get you started:

1. **Single Leg Stance:** Time to show off your one-legged stork move! Stand up nice and tall, feet hip-width apart. Now, shift your weight onto one leg while slightly lifting the other foot off the ground. Keep that core engaged and your eyes locked on a stable point. Try to hold the position for 30 seconds to 1 minute, then switch legs. It's like playing the statue game, but with balance skills!

2. **Heel-to-Toe Walk**: Prepare to walk the line! Position your feet in a heel-to-toe alignment, as if you're walking on a tightrope. Keep your gaze forward, arms out for balance, and start taking small steps. Each time you step, make sure your heel touches the toes of your other foot. See if you can walk in a straight line for 10 to 15 steps. Oh, and don't forget to turn around and do it all over again. It's like being a gymnast on a balance beam!

3. **Balance Board Exercises**: Time to get wobbly! Stand on a balance board or a wobble board with your feet hip-width apart. Engage that core of steel and keep your balance as the board tilts and shifts beneath you. Start with static balancing by holding the position for 30 seconds to 1 minute. Once you've mastered that, get ready for some dynamic moves. Shift your weight from side to side or try performing controlled squats on the balance board. It's like balancing on a floating platform!

4. **Yoga Tree Pose:** Welcome to the peaceful world of yoga! Stand tall, feet hip-width apart, and arms by your sides. Now, shift your weight onto one leg and place the sole of the other foot on the inner thigh or calf of the standing leg. Find your balance and bring your hands together at your chest in a prayer position. Can you hold that pose for 30 seconds to 1 minute? Then switch legs and repeat. You're like a majestic tree swaying in the wind!

5. **Tai Chi:** Prepare to channel your inner martial arts master! Tai Chi is all about slow, flowing movements and shifting body weight. It's like doing a dance with yourself! Practicing Tai Chi can improve your balance, coordination, and overall body awareness. You can find a local class or follow online tutorials to learn various Tai Chi exercises. Get ready to feel like a warrior!

Remember, start with exercises that match your current balance abilities and gradually progress as you become stronger and more stable. And safety first! Make sure you have a sturdy support nearby, like a wall or chair, just in case you need a little assistance. Balance exercises for 10 to 15 minutes, 3 or more days per week, will have you rocking those stability skills in no time!

WHICH MUSCLES DO I WORK OUT FIRST?

Hey there, fitness champs! Let's talk about the perfect workout order. You know, the way to organize those muscles and give them the VIP treatment they deserve. But hey, remember this is just a general guideline, so feel free to spice things up. Let's dive in!

Warm-up

First things first, warm-up time! Get that heart rate up and those muscles all warm and fuzzy. You can do some light jogging, jumping jacks, or even try some fancy dynamic stretches. It's like getting your body ready for the ultimate dance party!

Larger Muscle Groups

Now, let's tackle those larger muscle groups. They're like the big siblings of your muscles, so give them some early attention.

- Start with exercises that target your **legs and butt**. Think squats, lunges, step-ups, or leg presses. Work those lower body muscles while you still have all that energy. Go, go, power legs!
- Next, we move on to your **back.** It's time to show that back who's boss! Try some lat pulldowns and rows. These exercises hit those larger muscle groups in your back, and they'll benefit from your initial energy levels. Show them who's got your back!
- Now, it's time for your **chest**. You've got this! Wall push-ups, incline push-ups, or even the chest press machine can do the trick. These moves engage multiple muscles and can be performed effectively

early on in your routine. Show that chest some love and make it proud!

- Moving on to your **shoulders,** the crown of your upper body. Give them the attention they deserve! Overhead shoulder presses, lateral raises, front raises, and even halos can do the trick. These exercises require stability and control, so it's good to tackle them earlier in your workout. Give those shoulders a reason to shine!

Smaller Muscle Groups

Now, let's tackle the smaller muscle groups. They may be small, but they're still mighty!

- Time for those **arms**, baby! Bicep curls, triceps pushdowns, or triceps extensions are your new best friends. These are smaller muscle groups, so they can be worked after the larger ones have had their moment. Show those guns who's in charge!
- Lastly, let's not forget about the **core**. It's like the secret powerhouse of your body. Bird dogs, hip bridges, supine reverse marches, and planks are your go-to moves. They provide stability and support throughout various exercises, so they're perfect for the end of your workout. Show that core some love and let it be the foundation of your awesomeness!

Flexibility & Cooldown

- We're almost there, folks! Finish off with some static stretching exercises that target major muscle groups. It's like giving them a big ol' stretchy hug. Stretching improves flexibility and reduces muscle soreness.
- And don't forget the cool-down period! It's like gently lowering the curtain after a fantastic performance. Gradually lower your heart rate and let your body recover like the superstar it is.

Remember, this is just a general guideline, and you can always adjust the order to fit your preferences and needs.

LARGE LOWER BODY EXERCISES

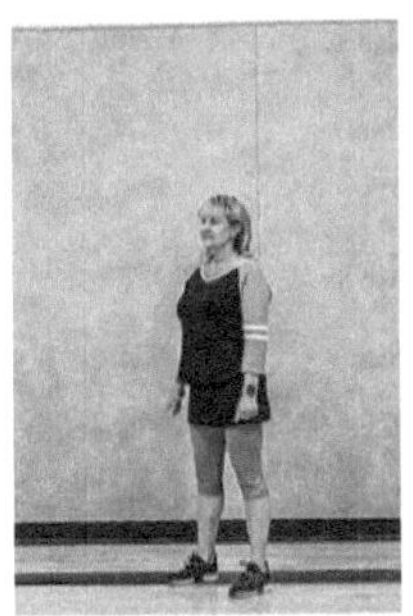 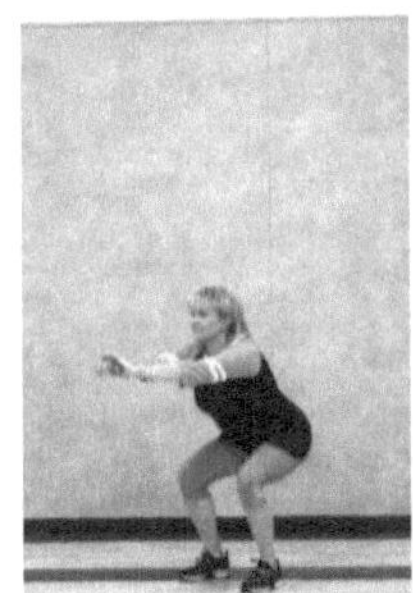

1. BODYWEIGHT SQUAT

Hey there, squat superstars! Get ready to tone those lower body muscles and show off your squatting skills. We're about to break down the bodyweight squat, the exercise that'll make your quads, hamstrings, and glutes go, "Wowza!" Here's how it's done:

1. Stand tall with your feet slightly wider than shoulder-width apart. You can position your feet parallel or give them a little turn-out, like you're ready to bust a move on the dance floor.
2. Engage that core power! Suck that belly button toward your spine, and keep that chest up and back straight throughout the whole squatting extravaganza. We want those muscles to be on point!

3. Now, let the squat party begin! Start by pushing your hips back and bending your knees. It's like you're lowering yourself into an imaginary chair. Get comfy!

4. As you descend, keep your weight on your heels and your knees aligned with your toes. We don't want any wobbly knees stealing the show!

5. Keep going until your thighs are parallel to the ground, or as low as your flexibility allows. Just remember, don't push those knees beyond your toes. We want everything to stay in the right place!

6. Take a moment to pause at the bottom of the squat. Enjoy the view down there. And when you're ready, press through those trusty heels to rise back up to the starting position. You're like a rising superstar, shining bright!

7. Don't forget to give your glutes some love! As you rise, squeeze those booty muscles like you're trying to crack a walnut. Engage that posterior chain, baby!

8. Keep the party going! Repeat the squat movement for 8-15 reps. Start with a comfortable range, and as you get the hang of it, go ahead and challenge yourself with more reps. You've got this!

And now, for some bonus tips to make your squats even more fabulous:

• Keep that head facing forward or slightly upward to maintain a neutral spine position. Look ahead and conquer those squats!

• Breathe, my friend, breathe! Inhale as you lower down into the squat, and exhale as you rise back up. It's like you're a squatting meditation master!

• For balance, you can extend your arms forward like Superman flying through the air, or place your hands on your hips like a confident superstar. Find the arm position that makes you feel like the squatting champion you are!

• Beginners or those with limited mobility, I've got a special chair edition just for you. Use a chair as a guide. Lower yourself until you lightly touch the chair with your booty, then rise back up. It's like a squatting safety net!

Remember, form is everything! We want to make those squats as effective as possible

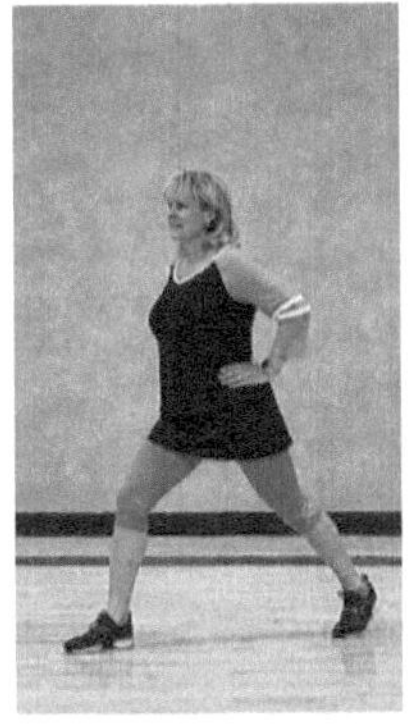 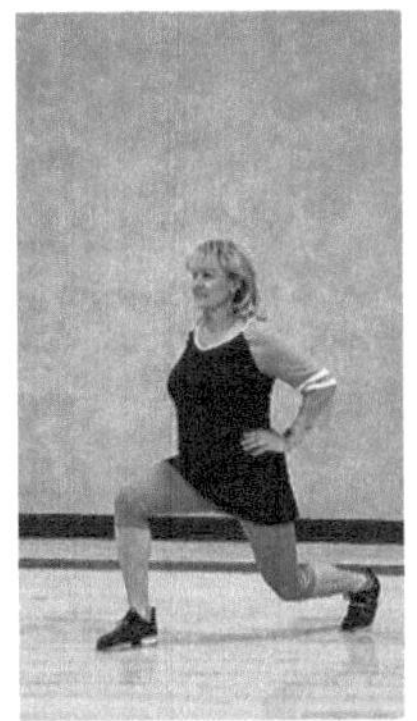

2. FRONT LUNGE

Hey there, lunge enthusiasts! Get ready to unleash your lower body strength with the mighty front lunge. It's a move that targets your quads, hamstrings, and glutes. Let's break it down step by step:

1. Stand tall and proud, feet hip-width apart. Engage that core like you're preparing for a tickle attack, and keep that chest up like you're wearing a badge of honor.
2. Now, it's time to take a bold step forward with your right foot. You want to make sure your stride is long enough to create a 90-degree angle at both your front and back knees when you lower into the lunge. Prepare to lunge like you mean it!
3. As you descend, bend those knees and drop those hips straight down toward the ground. It's like you're curtsying to the queen, but with way more power. Keep your front knee directly above your ankle, and let your back knee hover just above the ground. You've got this!
4. Keep that torso upright and avoid any wibbly-wobbly leaning. I want you to be the Tower of Lunge Power! So, no leaning too far forward or backward. Stay strong and steady.
5. Take a moment to pause at the bottom of the lunge, and then push through that front heel like you're about to jump off a trampoline. Rise back up to the starting position and engage those glutes and quadriceps. Show them who's boss!

6. Now, it's time to switch sides. Repeat the same powerful movement on the opposite side by stepping forward with your left foot. Alternate those lunges like you're a fancy dancer at a ball.

And here are some extra tips to make your lunges even more incredible:

• Keep it smooth and controlled. No bouncing or using momentum to perform the lunge.

• Engage that core like you're giving it a secret mission. It provides stability and protects your lower back.

• Watch those knees! Make sure your front knee stays in line with your ankle and doesn't extend past your toes.

• If you're new to the lunge game or need some balance support, you can start by doing lunges near a wall or holding onto a stable object. It's like having support until you feel comfortable going solo.

• You have options! You can choose to do all your reps on one leg before switching to the other leg, or you can alternate legs with each lunge. You can also hold dumbbells in each hand to up the ante. It's your lunge party, so you call the shots!

Remember, always listen to your body and adjust the intensity and range of motion according to your fitness level. I want you to feel strong and confident, not like a wobbly jellyfish.

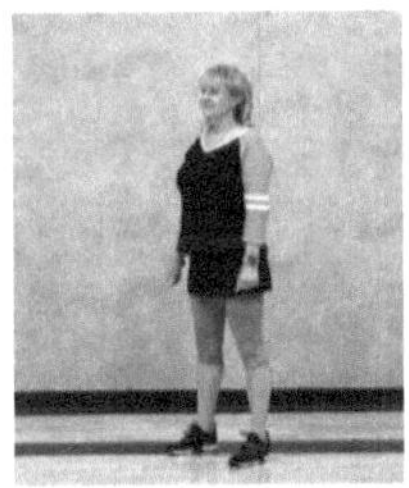 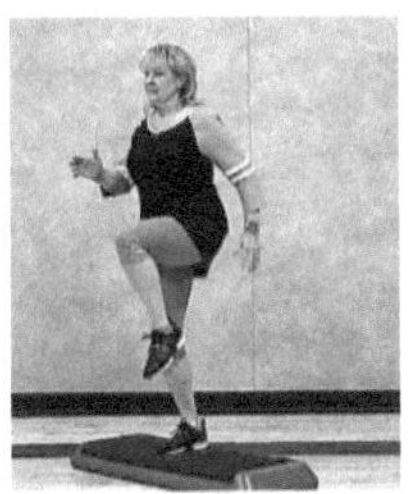

3. STEP- UPS

Get ready to level up your lower body strength with this fantastic body-weight exercise. We're talking quadriceps, hamstrings, and glutes getting their time in the spotlight. Let's break it down step by step:

1. Find yourself a stable platform or step. It could be your trusty stairs at home, a sturdy box, or even a bench at the gym. Make sure it's got your back!
2. Stand tall and proud, facing the step, with your feet hip-width apart. Engage that core like you're preparing for a tickle fight, and keep that chest up.
3. Lift your right foot like you're about to take it on a magical journey, and firmly place it on the step. Give that step a high-five with your entire foot, from heel to toe. We want a full-on foot connection!
4. Get ready to soar! Push through your right heel and engage those right glutes and quadriceps like they're your secret weapon. Lift your body up onto the step and straighten that right leg like a superhero in flight.
5. Now it's time for the left foot to join the party! Lift that foot off the ground and bring it up to the step, either next to your right foot or you can raise it up and bend your knee like you're doing a little dance move. You're making magic happen!
6. Ready to come back down to Earth? Step back down to the starting position with control and finesse. Lower your left foot first, followed by your right foot.

7. Keep the rhythm going! Repeat the movement, but this time lead with your left foot. Alternate between legs like a salsa dancer, keeping that energy flowing for the desired number of reps. You've got this!

And here are some extra tips to make your step-ups even more incredible:

• Keep it smooth and controlled, folks! We want precision, not chaos. Avoid dropping your foot onto the ground or relying on crazy momentum. Control is your superpower!

• Engage that core like you're guarding the secret recipe to the world's best ice cream. It provides stability and keeps your torso upright throughout the whole step-up show.

• Use those glutes and quadriceps to lift your body up and gracefully control the descent. They're like your trusted sidekicks, ready to support you on every step of the way.

• Safety first! Make sure that step or platform you're using is stable and secure. We don't want any unexpected adventures or mishaps. Safety is the name of the game!

• If you find the higher surfaces a bit challenging at first, no worries! Start with a lower step and gradually work your way up to higher platforms. Building strength and confidence is your journey!

As always, prioritize safety and use proper form during the exercise. Step it up, and show off those mighty lower body muscles

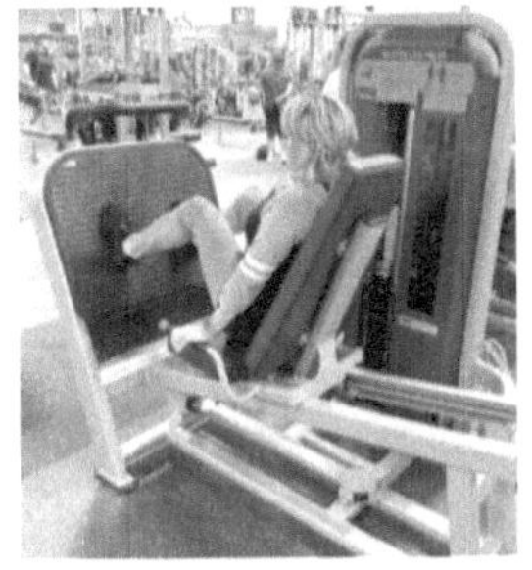 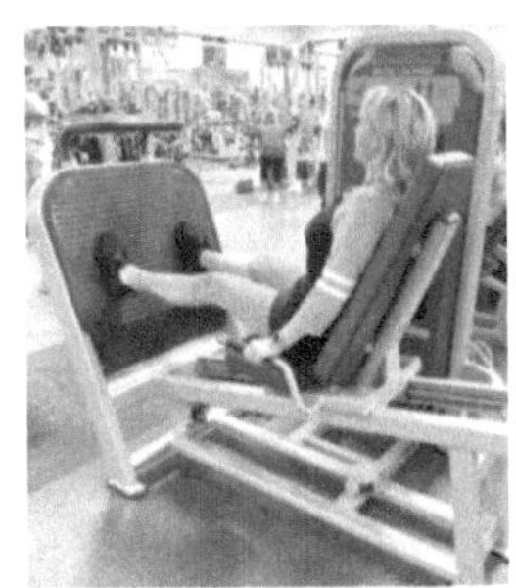

4. LEG PRESS MACHINE

Hey there, leg press adventurers! Get ready to give those lower body muscles a workout they won't forget. It's time to conquer the leg press machine and here's how to do it:

1. Take a seat in the machine like you're settling into a super comfy chair. Make sure your back is flat against the backrest, and your feet are placed on the resistance plate. Your toes should be pointing forward, and your heels should be flat on the plate. Get cozy!

2. It's time to engage those muscles and push like there's no tomorrow! Brace those abdominal muscles to stabilize your spine, and slowly exhale as you press through your heels and push that resistance away. Show that machine who's boss!

3. Watch out for those knees! We want to avoid any knee hyperextension. Keep those knees in check and maintain proper alignment. We're all about safety here!

4. Inhale deeply like you're taking a breath of fresh air, and slowly lower the weight back to the starting position. It's like you're bringing that resistance back home with control and finesse.

5. Let's keep the leg press party going! Repeat the movement for the desired number of repetitions according to your workout plan. You've got this! Your leg and butt muscles are going to thank you later.

6. Time to adjust and rest! Once you've completed your set, take a moment to adjust the weight if necessary. We want to make sure it's challenging but not overwhelming. And don't forget to take a well-deserved rest period before moving on to additional sets.

And there you have it, leg press conquerors! You now have the power to dominate that leg press machine with confidence and strength. Just remember, safety is key, so always listen to your body and adjust the weight and intensity according to your fitness level.

Now go forth, embrace those leg press challenges, and let your leg muscles shine. Crush those reps, take those rests, and enjoy the leg press adventure. You've got this, leg press champion!

LARGE MUSCLES -BACK EXERCISES

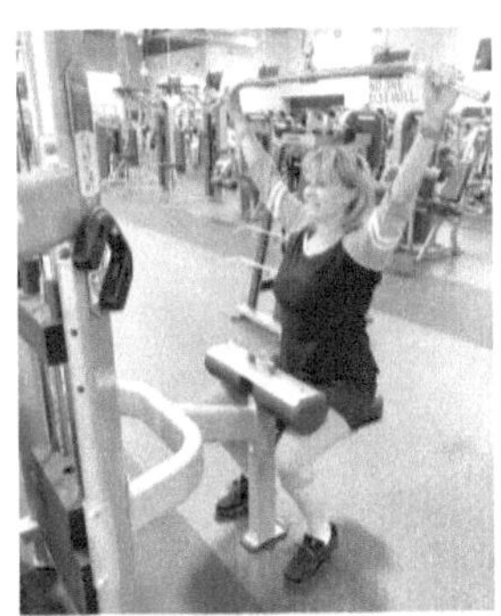 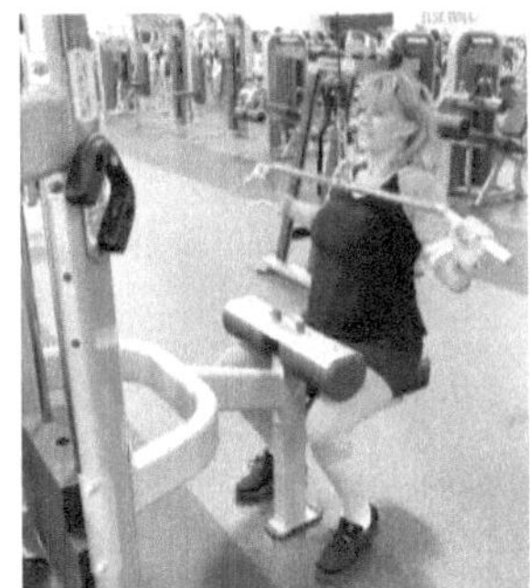

1. LAT PULL DOWN

Hey there, lat pulldown champs! Get ready to unleash your mighty lats and sculpt that back. It's time to conquer the lat machine pulldown and here's your step-by-step guide to rocking this exercise:

1. Adjust that machine to fit your awesome body! Set the seat height and knee pad to make sure you're sitting comfortably. We don't want any wedgies or awkward positions. Secure those thighs under the knee pad and get ready for action!

2. From a standing position, grab the wide bar attachment with an overhand grip, just a bit wider than your shoulders. Your palms should be facing forward, like you're about to give the lat machine a high-five. But be warned, it's a high-five with muscles!

3. Sit down while still holding the bar. Sit tall and proud! Keep that chest up, back straight, and maintain a slight arch in your lower back.

4. Time to unleash those shoulder blades! Before you start the movement, pull those shoulder blades down and back like you're trying to squeeze them together. Engage those back muscles like you're inviting them to the party.

5. Exhale as you pull that bar down towards your chest. Use those mighty lats and biceps to dominate the movement. Focus on squeezing your shoulder blades together like they're having a reunion.

6. Keep pulling that bar down like you're summoning all your strength. Bring it down to the level of your upper chest or just below. And remember, control your movement. No excessive swinging or momentum here!

7. Take a pause at the bottom of the movement and feel that contraction in your back muscles. It's like they're flexing and showing off. Embrace it!

8. Inhale deeply like you're breathing in energy and slowly release the bar. Let it return to the starting position in a controlled manner. Keep that back engaged throughout the exercise.

9. Repeat the movement for the desired number of reps. You're the director of your own destiny, so choose how many times you want to show off those lats and back muscles.

And here are some extra tips to make your lat pulldown even more super:

• Avoid any wild swinging or using your momentum to perform the exercise. It's all about those back muscles taking charge and controlling the movement.

• Keep those elbows pointed downward. No flaring them out to the sides like wings. We're not birds!

• Maintain a stable and neutral spine position. No leaning back or excessive arching of the lower back. We want stability and safety.

• If you're a beginner or feel like the weight is a bit too challenging, start with a lighter resistance. You're still in training, and with time and practice, you'll build that strength.

• And of course, always make sure the machine is set up properly and you're using the right weight for your abilities. Don't hesitate to ask a gym instructor for assistance if needed. We're all in this together!

So, get out there and conquer that lat machine pulldown like the true champions you are. Sculpt those lats, build that back, and let your strength shine.

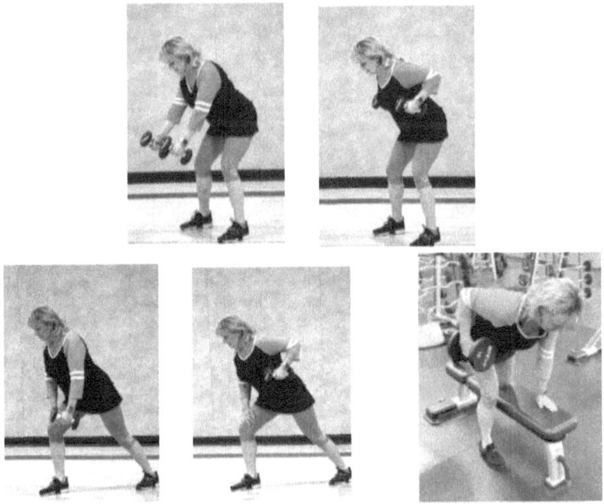

2. BENT OVER ROW / ONE ARM ROW

Alright, rowing warriors, get ready to conquer the bent-over row and unleash your mighty back muscles! It's time to row like a pro and build that strength. Here's your step-by-step guide to mastering the bent-over row:

1. Stand tall and proud with your feet shoulder-width apart. Grab hold of your weapon of choice - a barbell, dumbbells, or any other weight that tickles your fancy. Feel that power in your hands!

2. Now, it's time to unleash your rowing prowess. Hinge forward from your hips, keeping a slight bend in your knees. We're not doing the limbo here, but we're getting into position for some serious rowing action.

3. Imagine you're about to take flight. Keep that back straight and engage your core like you're wearing an invisible corset. We need that stability!

4. Let your arms hang naturally in front of you with a slight bend in your elbows. This is the starting position. You're like a coiled spring, ready to release that rowing power!

5. Exhale and pull that weight towards your lower chest or upper abdomen. Squeeze those shoulder blades together and bend those elbows

like your rowing. Activate those back muscles and show them who's boss!

6. Feel that contraction in your back as you reach the top of the movement. Hold it for a moment and let the world marvel at your back muscles. It's like your back is saying, "Look at me now!"

7. Inhale deeply and slowly lower the weight back down to the starting position. Keep that control. We don't want any wild swinging or dropping of weights. You're the picture of grace and control.

8. Repeat the movement for 8-15 reps. It's your rowing show! You're the star of this exercise. Show those back muscles who's the boss in town!

And here are some extra tips to make your bent-over row even more epic:

• Don't round your back or let those shoulders roll forward. Maintain a strong and stable posture throughout. No slouching allowed!

• Activate that core like it's the key to unlocking your powers. Engage those muscles to provide stability and support for your lower back. We need that rock-solid foundation!

• Keep those elbows close to your body as you row. We don't want any flailing arms or chicken wing action. It's all about that precision and control.

• If you're using a barbell, feel free to experiment with different grip widths. Find the one that targets your back muscles just right.

• Start with a weight that challenges you but still allows you to maintain proper form. As you become stronger and more proficient, feel free to increase the resistance and take your rowing to the next level.

• And if you have any lower back issues or limitations, fear not! You can unleash the power of the ONE ARM ROW. Rest your non-working hand and knee on a bench or on your knee for added support.

Row like the wind!

LARGE MUSCLES : CHEST

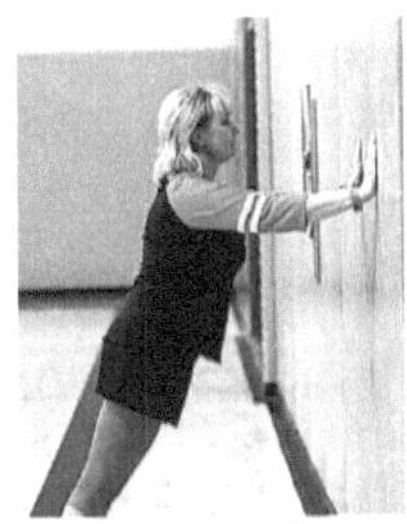 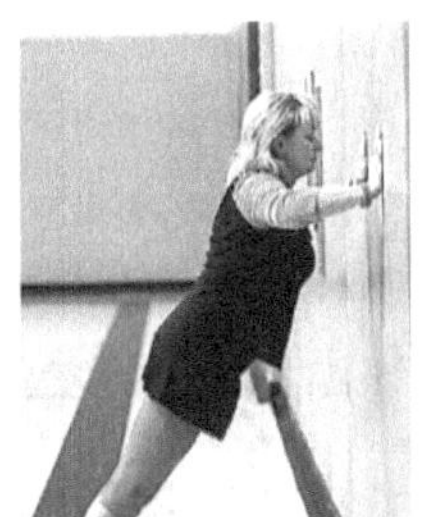

1. WALL PUSH - UP:

Alright, my aspiring wall push-up champs, get ready to build some serious chest, shoulder, and arm muscles. We're about to embark on a journey of wall-pushing awesomeness! Follow these steps, and you'll be a wall push-up pro in no time.

1. Find yourself a trusty wall. Stand about arm's length away from it, giving it some personal space. We don't want to invade its wall-ness, right? Keep your feet shoulder-width apart, and extend your arms in front of you, resting your hands on the wall at shoulder height.
2. Lean forward, my brave wall conquerors, and place your hands flat against the wall. Your hands should be slightly wider than shoulder-width apart, like you're about to give the wall a friendly high-five. Show that wall some love!
3. Now, my wall-pushing warriors, it's time to engage your core like it's a secret weapon. Keep that body straight and sturdy,

4. Get ready for the descent! Lower your chest towards the wall by bending your elbows. Keep that back straight and show the wall who's boss. We want a controlled movement here, no crashing into the wall like a bull in a china shop.

5. Keep going, my unstoppable wall push-up masters! Lower your body until your nose or chin comes close to the wall. Look at you, forming a perfect 90-degree angle with those elbows. You're like a geometry genius!

6. Take a brief pause, catch your breath, and get ready for the ascent. Push yourself back up by straightening your arms, like you're gently nudging the wall away. Exhale and extend those elbows, returning to the starting position. You're defying gravity with every push!

7. Repeat the exercise for 8-15 reps. Aim for the number of repetitions that feels challenging yet doable. You're in control of this wall-pushing extravaganza!

And here are some additional tips to make your wall push-ups even more epic:

• Focus on maintaining proper form, my wall warriors. Keep that body straight, engage that core, and don't let those hips sag or your back round. We want great posture!

• Start at a comfortable distance from the wall, my beginner champions. As you grow stronger and more confident, feel free to step back and increase the difficulty. You're like an unstoppable force of wall-pushing power!

So, with regular practice and a touch of determination, you'll build strength in your chest, shoulders, and arms like never before. Let the wall-pushing journey begin!

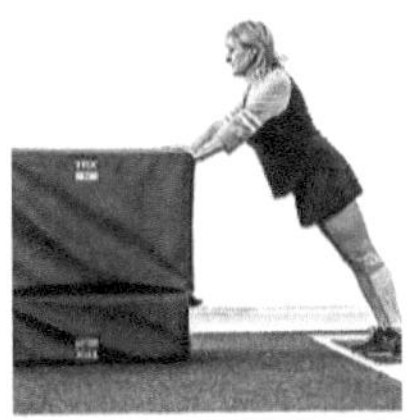 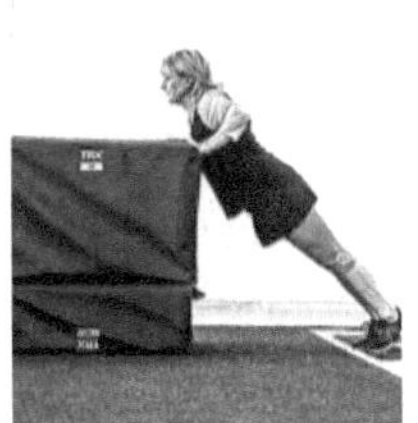

2. INCLINE PUSH- UP

Alright, my aspiring incline push-up champions, it's time to elevate your fitness game! Get ready to conquer those elevated surfaces with your push-up prowess. Follow these steps, and you'll be rocking incline push-ups like a boss:

1. Find yourself a trusty elevated surface. Look for a bench, a step, a counter or even a sturdy platform that can handle your mighty body weight. We need something stable and reliable for this epic push-up adventure. No wobbly surfaces allowed!

2. Position yourself like a push-up superstar. Stand facing the elevated surface, and place your hands on the edge slightly wider than shoulder-width apart. Your palms should be facing downward, ready to push you to greatness. Step back, extending your arms and keeping those feet together. You're about to take flight!

3. Set your body position and make sure your body forms a straight line from your head to your heels, just like a plank. Engage those core muscles like they're secret weapons, and maintain a neutral spine throughout the exercise. You're a plank master!

4. It's time to descend, my mighty push-up pros! Slowly lower your chest toward the edge of the elevated surface, maintaining that alignment. Inhale through your nose, and keep those elbows close to your sides like they're your loyal sidekicks. No elbow flaring or shoulder shrugging allowed! We want controlled and powerful movements.

5. Now, it's time to rise, my incredible incline push-up champions! Press through your hands and extend those arms like you're pushing away

any doubts or limitations. Feel your chest, shoulders, and triceps as you exhale through your mouth. Keep that core engaged, maintain control, and rise to greatness!

6. Repeat the epic movement! Perform 8-15 reps. Remember to focus on maintaining proper form and control throughout the exercise. You're in charge of this incline push-up adventure, and nothing can stop you!

Incline push-ups are a modified version of traditional push-ups. They're like the training wheels for regular push-ups. They help build strength in your chest, shoulders, and triceps while also engaging those powerful core muscles. As you become more comfortable and stronger, you can gradually decrease the height of the elevated surface. It's like removing those training wheels and unleashing your full potential!

So, my mighty incline push-up warriors, go forth and conquer those elevated surfaces. Embrace the challenge, and show them what you're made of! Let the incline push-up journey begin!

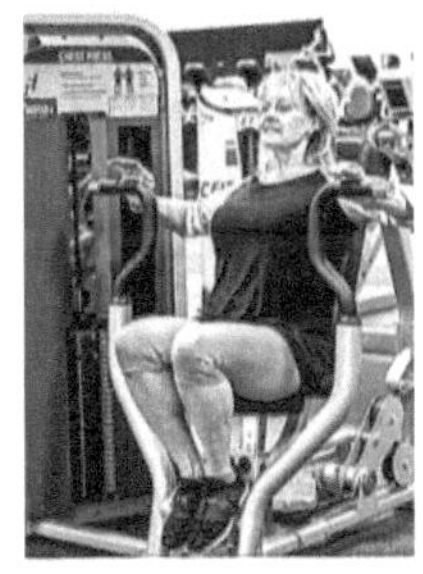 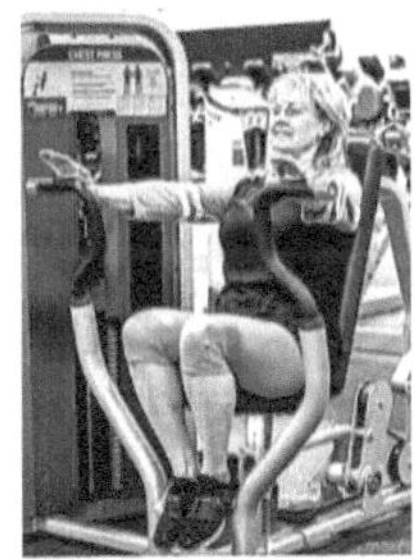

3. CHEST PRESS MACHINE

Alright, my fellow chest press enthusiasts, get ready to flex those pecs and conquer that machine! Here's your ticket to chest muscle greatness with a step-by-step guide on how to use a chest press machine:

1. First things first, let's get cozy with that machine. Adjust the seat height and backrest to fit your awesome body. We want those handles or grips to be right around chest height when you're seated. No need to strain or stretch. It's all about that perfect fit!
2. Take a seat on the machine and make yourself comfortable. Plant that back of yours firmly against the backrest like you mean it. You're in command here!
3. Get a grip, but not just any grip. Grasp those handles or grips with an overhand grip, slightly wider than shoulder-width apart. Your palms should be facing forward, ready to push some serious chest power. Show those handles who's boss!
4. Check your angles. We want those elbows at approximately a 90-degree angle when your hands are at chest level. This is your starting position, the launching pad for chest greatness!
5. Exhale, summon your chest muscles, and unleash that power! Push the handles or grips forward, extending your arms in front of you as if you are repelling a swarm of pesky mosquitos. Feel that chest muscle activation, my fellow pec warriors!
6. Inhale and bring it back. Slowly and gracefully, bend those elbows and bring the handles back to the starting position. Feel that controlled

motion and keep that chest muscle tension in check. You're the maestro of this chest press symphony!

7. Repeat, my fellow chest press champions! Perform 8-15 reps, always keeping that proper form in mind. It's all about quality over quantity.

Additional tips to keep you ahead of the chest press game:

• Keep that back firmly against the backrest throughout the entire exercise. We want stability and support for your magnificent spine.

• No need for jerky movements. Embrace that smooth and controlled motion like a chest press maestro.

• Engage that core of yours like it's your secret weapon. It provides stability and prevents any excessive arching or rounding of your lower back. Your core is your trusty sidekick!

• Squeeze those shoulder blades together like you're trying to hold a secret treasure. This activates your chest muscles and ensures maximum pec power.

• We don't want those elbows locking out completely at the end of the movement. Let's keep that tension on your chest muscles.

Start with a weight that suits your strength, and gradually increase the resistance as you become stronger and more proficient. Remember, it's all about that proper form and progression!

Now go forth, my magnificent chest press warriors, and conquer that machine like the chest muscle champions you are! Show those pecs who's boss!

LARGE MUSCLES – SHOULDERS

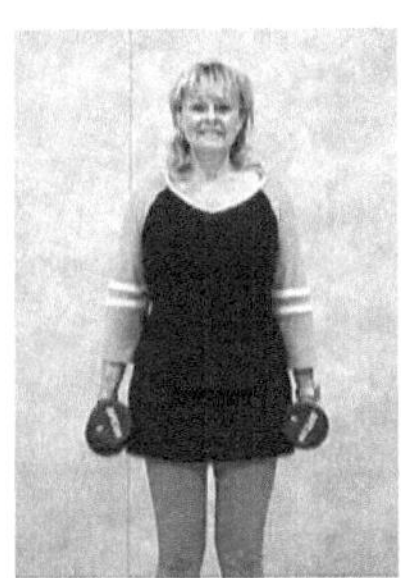 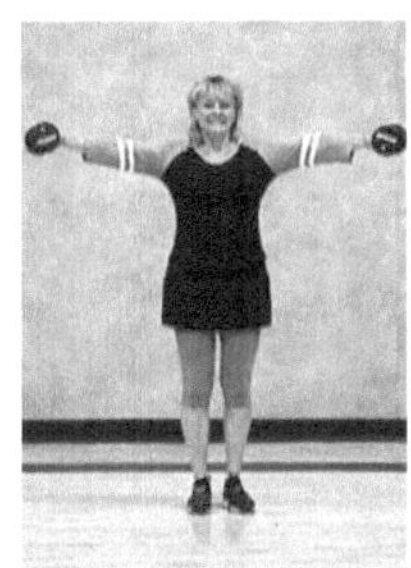

1. LATERAL RAISES:

Listen up, shoulder warriors! We're about to conquer those mid and posterior deltoids with an exercise that's gonna make your shoulders say, "Wow, you're raising the bar!" Let's dive into the step-by-step guide on how to do lateral raises:

1. Stand tall and proud! Plant those feet shoulder-width apart and grab a dumbbell in each hand. If you don't have dumbbells, don't worry! You can get creative and use resistance bands or even pretend you're lifting weights. Imagination is the key!

2. Let those arms hang loose by your sides, palms facing your body. This is your starting position, the calm before the shoulder storm.

3. Engage that core like it's a shield, keeping your back straight and maintaining a slight bend in those elbows. We don't want those elbows to turn into noodle arms!

4. Exhale and let the lifting begin! Raise those dumbbells out to the sides, away from your body. Keep those arms straight or slightly bent at the elbows, like a graceful bird spreading its wings. Go until your arms are parallel to the floor or slightly below shoulder level. You'll be rockin' a cool "T" shape with your body. Embrace it!

5. Hold it right there! Take a moment to squeeze those shoulder muscles like you're trying to catch a slippery watermelon seed between them.

6. Inhale and lower those dumbbells back down to the starting position with the grace of a feather. Control is the name of the game. Don't let gravity boss you around!

7. Repeat, repeat, and repeat some more! Perform 8-15 reps, always focusing on maintaining that proper form and control. You're the captain of this shoulder ship!

Additional tips to elevate your lateral raises:

• Keep it smooth Avoid any wild swinging or jerking movements. This exercise is all about that controlled motion.

• It's all about the shoulders, baby! Focus on using those shoulder muscles to lift those dumbbells, no cheating allowed! Other body parts are just spectators in this shoulder show.

• We don't want to overdo it. Lift those dumbbells until your arms are parallel to the floor or slightly below shoulder level. Let's protect those precious shoulder joints!

• Spice it up, shoulder style! You can slightly vary the angle of your arms during the exercise to target different parts of those shoulder muscles. For example, move your arms diagonally. Let's hit 'em from all angles!

• If you're new to the shoulder game or find dumbbells too heavy, start with lighter weights or use resistance bands. You'll build that shoulder strength in no time!

Now, go forth and conquer those lateral raises like the shoulder champions you are! Show those deltoids who's boss and let your shoulders shine bright like the stars!

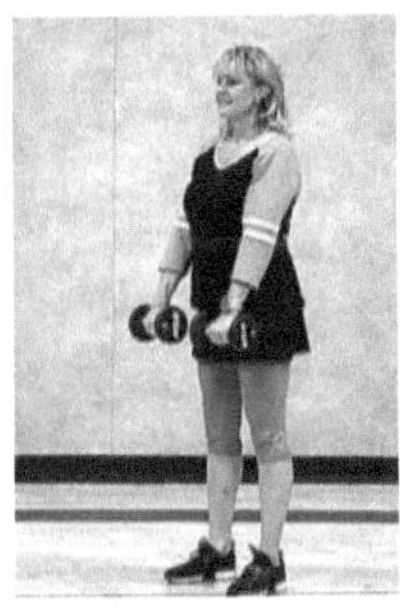 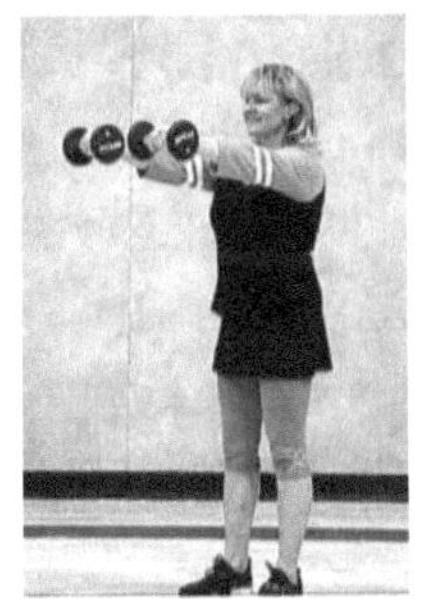

2. FRONT DUMBBELL RAISES:

Alrighty, shoulder superstars! It's time to give those front delts a little love with a move that'll have you saying, "Hey, shoulders, watch me raise the bar!" Let's dive into the step-by-step guide on how to do dumbbell front raises:

1. Stand tall and proud! Plant those feet shoulder-width apart and grab a dumbbell in each hand. Remember, if you don't have dumbbells, you can always get creative and use water bottles, soup cans, or even two pineapples! Let's get fruity with it!

2. Let those arms hang in front of you, palms facing your body. This is your starting position, the calm before the shoulder storm.

3. Engage that core like it's protecting your secret stash of snacks, keeping your back straight and maintaining a slight bend in those elbows. We don't want those elbows to turn into spaghetti noodles!

4. Get ready to rock and raise! Exhale and lift one or both dumbbells directly in front of you. Keep those arms straight or slightly bent at the elbows. Your goal is to lift those weights until they reach shoulder height. We're going for the Goldilocks zone here, not too high, not too low, just right!

5. Hold it right there! Take a moment to squeeze those front deltoid muscles. Enjoy the moment of front delt domination!

6. Inhale and lower those dumbbells back down to the starting position gracefully. We're all about that controlled descent. Show gravity who's boss!

7. Repeat, repeat, and switch it up! If you're using one dumbbell at a time, alternate between arms like you're passing a hot potato. Keep those front delts on their toes!

Additional tips to elevate your dumbbell front raises:

• Smooth and steady wins the race! Avoid any wild swinging or jerking motions. We're all about that controlled movement here.

• Let those front delts shine! Focus on using those shoulder muscles to lift those dumbbells, no shortcuts allowed! Other body parts can sit back and enjoy the front delt show.

• Keep those wrists straight because we don't want any wobbly wrists stealing the spotlight.

• Stand tall, shoulders relaxed, and chest up throughout the exercise. Good posture is the secret ingredient to super shoulders!

• If you're finding it challenging with heavier dumbbells, start with lighter weights and work your way up. Rome wasn't built in a day, and neither were your shoulders!

Now go forth and conquer those dumbbell front raises like the front delt heroes you are! Show those muscles who's boss and let your shoulders steal the spotlight. Keep raising the bar

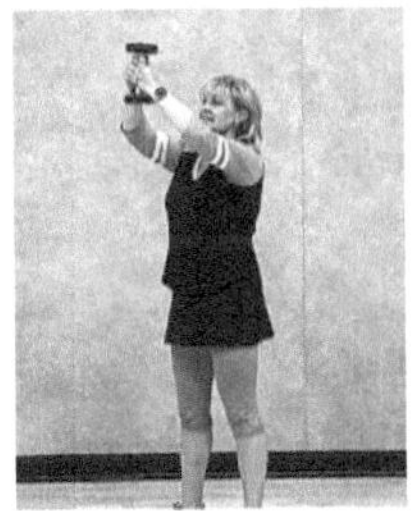 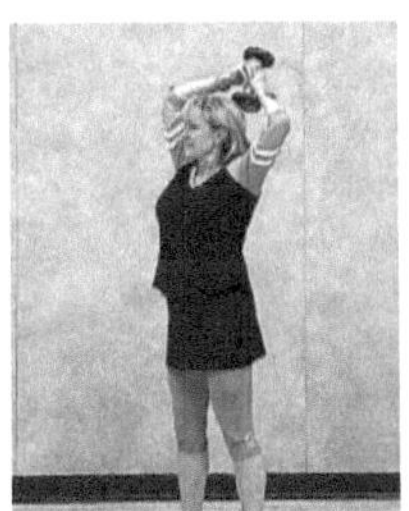

3. HALO:

Alright, shoulder champs, get ready to rock the halo exercise and give those delts a heavenly workout! Here's your step-by-step guide to mastering the halo:

1. Stand tall with your feet shoulder-width apart, like a majestic statue guarding the entrance to the shoulder temple. Grab a dumbbell or kettlebell by the handle with both hands, and hold it in front of your chest. We're about to embark on a divine journey!
2. Engage that core like you're preparing to withstand an asteroid impact. Keep your back straight with good posture. No slouching allowed!
3. Lift that weight slightly away from your body, positioning it just above your forehead. You're about to wear a weighty halo with style!
4. Take a deep breath and exhale with confidence. Now, let's start moving that weight in a circular motion around your head. Imagine you're painting a glorious halo around yourself, but with a weight instead of a brush.
5. As you trace that celestial circle, keep those elbows slightly bent and maintain control. We're not twirling a lasso here, folks. No swinging or drifting allowed! Keep that weight close to your body like it's your celestial companion.
6. Complete a full circle, bringing the weight back to the starting position above your forehead. You've just painted a magnificent halo masterpiece in the air. Michelangelo would be proud!
7. But wait, the divine journey isn't over! It's time to reverse direction and perform the halo exercise in the opposite direction. We want a

symmetrical heavenly glow, after all. Complete that second circle with grace and precision.

8.   Repeat, repeat, and repeat! Keep going for your desired number of repetitions in each direction. The more halos you create, the stronger those shoulder muscles will become. You're on your way to shoulder sainthood!

Additional tips to make your halos shine brighter:

• Slow and steady wins the celestial race! Keep the movement controlled and deliberate throughout the exercise. No need for cosmic speed here.

• Focus on engaging those shoulder and shoulder blade muscles as you perform the halo.

• If you're using a heavier weight, pay extra attention to your grip and ensure you have a firm hold.

• Start with a lighter weight or even practice the movement without weight to get the hang of it. We're all about building strength and confidence on this divine journey.

• Listen to your shoulders and neck.

Now go forth, my shoulder angels, and embrace the halo exercise with grace and strength. Let those delts shine bright like celestial beacons. Your shoulders are reaching for the heavens!

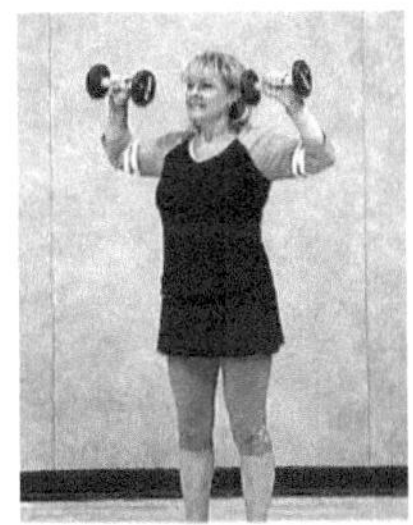 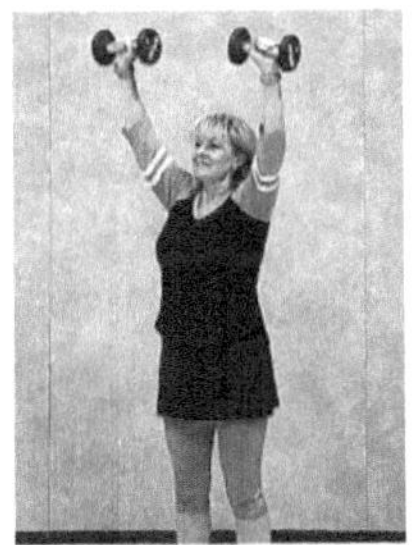

4. OVERHEAD SHOULDER PRESS:

Get ready to lift your shoulders to new heights with the overhead press! It's time to give those deltoids a workout they won't forget. Here's your step-by-step guide:

1. Stand tall like a champion, feet shoulder-width apart, holding your weapons of choice: a barbell, dumbbells, kettlebells, or even resistance bands. You're about to unleash the fury on those shoulders!
2. Engage your core. Keep that back straight, and don't forget to bend your knees slightly. We want a solid foundation here!
3. If you've chosen the mighty barbell, grab it with a grip slightly wider than shoulder-width apart. Palms facing forward, like you're about to conquer the world. If you're wielding dumbbells or kettlebells, hold them with an overhand grip, palms still facing forward, and your elbows bent at a perfect 90-degree angle. This is your starting position, and you're looking fierce!
4. Take a deep breath and brace yourself. It's time to exhale and push those weights directly overhead. Extend your arms fully, like you're lifting the roof off a secret lair. Keep your head neutral, no excessive tilting back here!
5. Halt! Freeze! Hold that victorious pose for a moment at the top, squeezing those shoulder muscles like a vise. You're the conqueror of deltoids!

6. Inhale and lower those weights back down to the starting position. Take your time, control the movement, and let your elbows bend as your hands gracefully return to the front of your shoulders.
7. Ready to unleash your power again? Repeat the movement for 8-15 reps. Those shoulders won't know what hit them!

Additional tips to keep your overhead press on point:

• Maintain a posture that says, "I'm the hero of this shoulder show!" No excessive arching or rounding of your lower back. Stand tall and stable throughout the exercise.

• Engage that core, your secret weapon for stability and support during the overhead press. It's like having a trusty sidekick by your side!

• Don't lock out those elbows at the top of the movement. We want to keep those shoulder muscles engaged and under tension.

• If you're feeling adventurous with dumbbells or kettlebells, try different grip positions. You can go for a neutral grip, where your palms face each other, to give those shoulder muscles a fresh challenge.

• Start with a weight that allows you to maintain proper form, and gradually increase the resistance as your strength grows.

Remember, form is everything! If you're new to the overhead press or have any concerns, it's always wise to seek guidance from a qualified fitness professional. Safety first!

SMALLER MUSCLES – ARMS

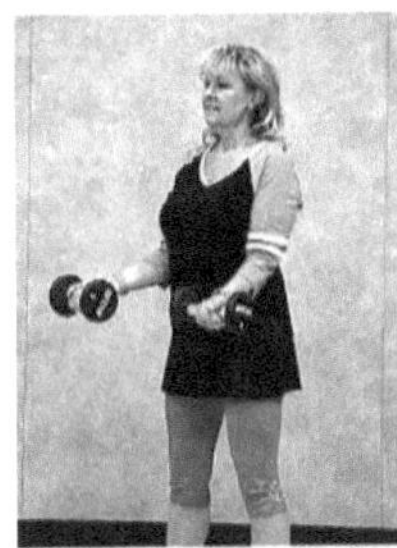 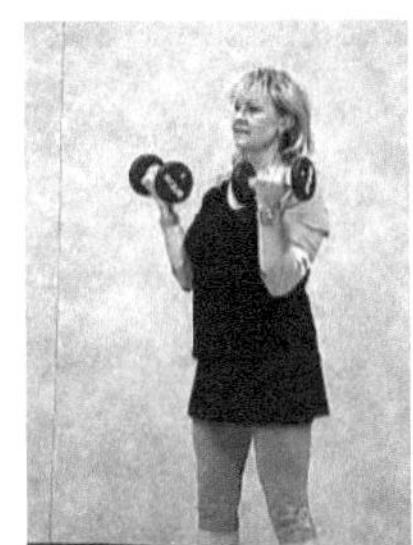

1. BICEPS CURLS:

Get ready to flex those guns with the bicep curl! We're about to pump up those biceps like there's no tomorrow. Here's your step-by-step guide:

1. Stand tall with your feet shoulder-width apart. Grab those dumbbells and let your arms hang naturally by your sides. Palms facing forward, because we're ready to show off those guns!
2. Engage that core like a fortress, keeping that back straight and those knees slightly bent. We need a solid foundation for this bicep extravaganza!
3. Take a deep breath and prepare for lift-off. Exhale as you slowly lift one or both dumbbell(s) toward your shoulder. Bend the elbow(s), but keep the upper arm(s) steady as a rock. We want those forearms to do all the heavy lifting!
4. Keep pumping that iron until your forearm is standing tall at attention. Your biceps should be fully contracted, and you should feel that glorious squeeze. Squeeze it like you mean it!

5. Inhale like a bicep master and gently lower the dumbbell back down to the starting position. Control is the name of the game here. Extend that elbow, and let your forearm straighten out.

6. Repeat the movement with the opposite arm. Alternate between those arms for 8-15 reps. Those biceps won't know what hit them!

Additional tips to keep those biceps in check:

• Stay in control. No swinging or wild motions allowed. We want slow and steady curls, not a bicep circus.

• It's all about those biceps, baby! Focus on using those muscles to lift the dumbbells, not your back or any other sneaky body parts.

• Keep those wrists neutral, like a cool secret agent. No funky bending or arching of the wrists. We want to keep those biceps in the spotlight.

• We're all about the biceps here, so no leaning back or using your back and shoulders to lift the weight. Keep that upper body stable and let those biceps steal the show!

• If you're just starting out or feeling like a bicep newbie, start with lighter weights and work your way up. We're building bicep confidence, one curl at a time.

Remember, it's all about the biceps, baby! Form and control are key, so make sure you're doing those curls with finesse.. Now go out there and rock those biceps

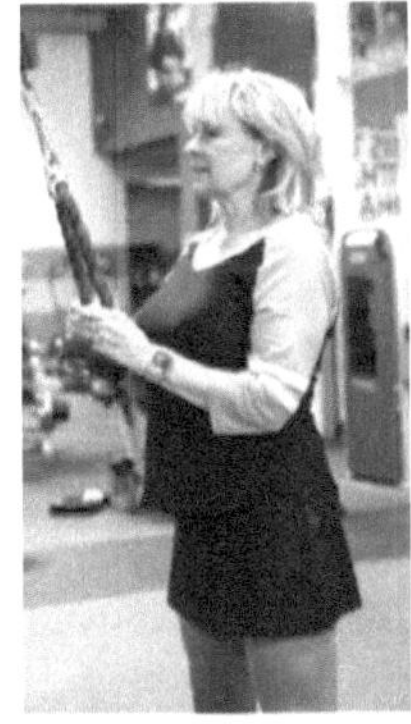 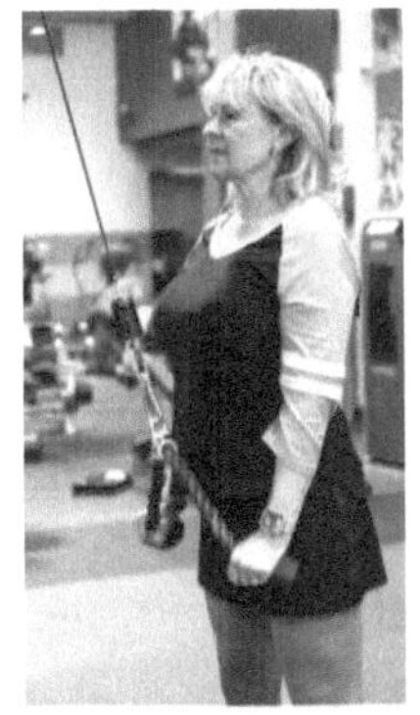

2. TRICEPS PUSH – DOWNS:

Alright, triceps warriors, it's time to get those "bye-bye arm flaps" in check with the tricep's pushdown – the secret sauce for sculpting the back of those upper arms!

1. First things first – picture yourself facing a cable machine, ready to take on those triceps! Adjust that pulley thingy to the right height so your arms can fully extend when you're standing tall.

2. Now, get a grip – literally! Grab that straight bar or rope attachment with your mighty hands, shoulder-width apart, and palms facing down. We're about to give those triceps a good talking to!

3. Make sure your elbows are chillin' by your sides and slightly bent   this is your starting position, and you're already looking like a pro!

4. Engage that core of yours and keep your back straight, like you're showing off to the world how awesome you are. And don't forget to keep a teeny bend in those knees.

5. Time to push it! Exhale as you extend your arms down, pushing that bar or rope towards your mighty thighs. Straighten those arms like you mean business, but keep those elbows close and steady by your sides. No wobbling allowed!

6. At the bottom of the move, pause and give those triceps a squeeze – show 'em some love, and they'll thank you later!

7. Now, take a deep breath and slowly return to the starting position. Let the bar or rope rise back up, resisting the weight like a boss.

8. Rinse and repeat to do more reps.

Additional tips to keep those triceps in check:
- Keep that control, team! No swinging or using momentum – it's all about being a triceps mastermind!
- And remember, keep those wrists neutral – no bending or arching like Gumby!
- Relax those shoulders and let go of any tension – we want you feeling good and confident!
- Oh, and for all you rope attachment peeps – have some fun with it! Try different hand positions like a neutral grip or overhand grip to target those triceps from all angles!
- Start with a weight that's just right for you – one that allows you to show off perfect form within 8-15 reps! Gradually increase the resistance as you become stronger and more awesome!
- Now, if you don't have a fancy cable machine, no worries! Resistance bands to the rescue! Securely anchor that band and get pushin'!

Alright, my triceps heroes, you've got the power to rock this exercise like nobody's business! Show off those strong triceps and get ready to flex those arms with pride! Let's do this!

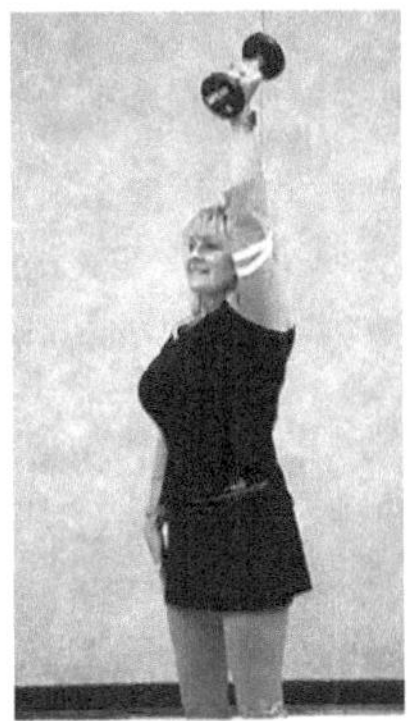 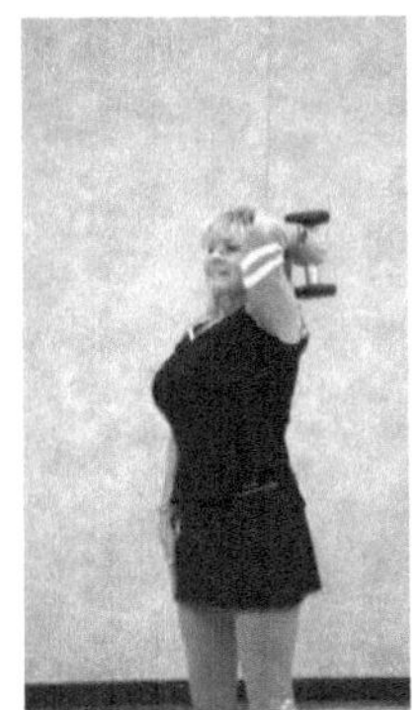

3. TRICEPS EXTENSION:

Alright, let's get those triceps in shape! We're about to tackle the triceps extensions, the exercise that will have those flabby arms waving goodbye. Here's the scoop on how to do it:

1. Stand tall with your feet shoulder-width apart, and grab a trusty dumbbell in one hand. Extend that arm overhead so the dumbbell is right above your shoulder. This is your starting position, and you're ready to rock!
2. Engage that core like you're about to save the world, and keep that back straight with a slight bend in those knees. We need a solid foundation for this triceps extravaganza!
3. Take a deep breath and get ready to unleash those triceps. Inhale as you slowly lower the dumbbell behind your head, bending that elbow. Keep that upper arm locked in place, nice and close to your head. Your forearm should be parallel to the floor or just a smidge below.
4. Exhale and extend that arm like you're showing off your triceps to the world. Raise that dumbbell back up, feeling the power in those triceps. Give them a good squeeze at the top of the movement, like you're saying, "Look at these guns!"
5. Take a moment to soak in the triceps glory at the top, and then get ready to do it all over again. Repeat the movement for 8-15 reps. We're sculpting those triceps, one extension at a time!

6. Oh, and don't forget to switch to the other arm after you've given the first arm its moment in the spotlight. Those triceps deserve equal attention!

Additional tips to keep those triceps in tip-top shape:

• Slow and steady wins the triceps race! Keep those movements controlled and avoid any swinging or wild motions. We're focused on targeting those triceps, not putting on a triceps circus!

• It's all about those triceps, baby! Concentrate on using those muscles to extend your arm, and leave the rest of your body out of it. No cheating allowed!

• Watch those wrists. Keep them in a neutral position and avoid any crazy bending or arching. We're sculpting triceps, not contorting our wrists!

• If you're feeling adventurous, you can use both hands to hold a dumbbell or an E-Z bar and give those triceps a double dose of love. Just make sure you maintain good form and control.

• If you're lifting a heavier weight, you may want to stabilize your non-working arm by placing it on your hip or giving it a supportive hand. We're all about balance and safety here!

• Start with a weight that challenges you but still allows you to maintain proper form. As you become stronger, gradually increase the resistance. We're building triceps of steel!

So there you have it—your ticket to triceps greatness. Form, control, and a whole lot of triceps power. Now go out there and wave those sculpted triceps with pride!

CORE EXERCISES

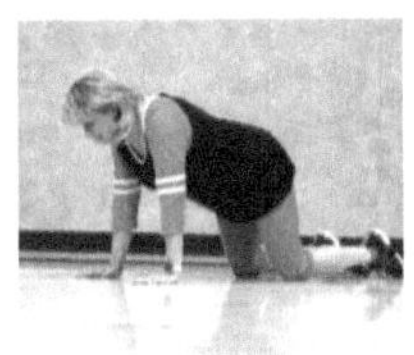 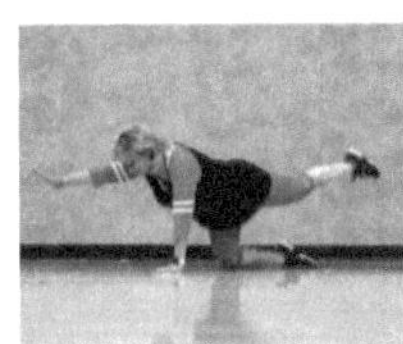

1. BIRD DOG:

Alrighty, let's fly like a bird and strengthen that core with the bird dog exercise! Get ready to unleash your inner bird and feel those muscles in action. Here's how to do it:

1. Get down on all fours. Place your hands directly under your shoulders and your knees right under your hips. Keep that back of yours in a sweet neutral position—no arching or rounding, we want it just right.
2. Time to engage that core. Draw your belly button in towards your spine, activating those abs and stabilizing that torso.
3. Extend your right arm straight forward, reaching it out in front of you like you're trying to give a high-five to a friendly bird. At the same time, extend your left leg straight back, reaching it out behind you. Keep that arm and leg in line with your torso..
4. We're all about straight lines here, so make sure you maintain a perfect line from your fingertips to your toes. No sagging or twisting in those hips or shoulders. Keep that body parallel to the floor, as if you're soaring through the sky.

5. Hold this position for a few seconds and feel that core stability. Imagine you're a bird gracefully gliding through the air. Keep that core engaged and stay strong!

6. Gently lower your arm and leg back down to the starting position, like a bird returning to its cozy nest.

7. Time to switch sides and give the other arm and leg a turn. Extend your left arm forward and your right leg back. Show off your balancing skills and feel those core muscles in action.

8. Keep alternating sides, just like a bird showing off its fancy aerial moves. Fly from side to side for your desired number of repetitions or time. You've got this!

Some extra tips to keep your bird dog game strong:

• Be the master of control! Keep those movements smooth and steady, and avoid any jerking or wild swings. We want to be graceful birds, not flapping feathers in a frenzy.

• Focus on stability and balance. Engage that core like you're preparing for a balancing act on a tightrope. Keep your body aligned and maintain that straight line.

• Say no to back arches and rounded spines. Keep that back of yours neutral and straight. No bird wants a wonky posture!

• Breathe, my feathered friend. Inhale and exhale with ease and grace. We want controlled breaths, just like a bird enjoying the breeze.

• If you're finding it a bit tricky to maintain your balance, start by extending just your arm or leg and work your way up to the full bird dog. Rome wasn't built in a day, and neither was your bird dog prowess!

• Feeling extra adventurous? Spice things up by holding the extended position for a longer time or add some resistance bands or ankle weights. You'll level up your bird dog game in no time!

So there you have it—the bird dog exercise. Modify it to fit your fitness level and make it a regular part of your core or full-body workout routine. Embrace your inner bird and soar to new heights of core strength!

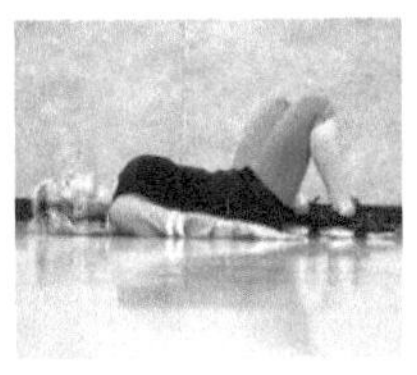 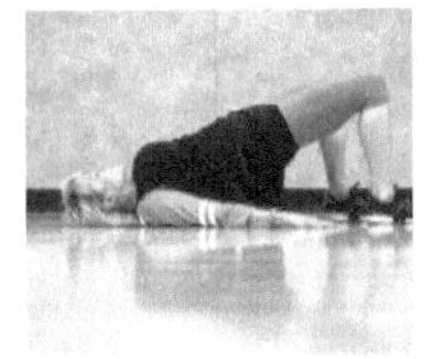

2. HIP BRIDGE:

Alrighty, let's bridge those hips and build some booty power! Get ready to work those glutes, hamstrings, and lower back like a pro. Here's how to perform the hip bridge exercise:

1. Get comfy! Lie flat on your back on a squishy exercise mat or a nice and cozy surface. Bend those knees of yours and plant your feet firmly on the ground, about hip-width apart. Let your arms rest comfortably by your sides, palms facing down.

2. Engage that core. Draw your belly button in towards your spine, activating those abs and stabilizing your entire torso. You're a core-stabilizing superstar!

3. Time to press those feet into the ground like you mean it! Push through your mighty heels and lift those hips off the floor, squeezing those glutes with all your might. We're aiming for a straight line from your knees to your shoulders, so don't go overboard and lift too high—no rocket launches here!

4. Hold it! Pause at the top of the movement and embrace the glute squeeze. Squeeze those buns of steel and maintain a stable and strong position.

5. Slowly lower those hips back down to the starting position, under control. No sudden drops or crazy falls—keep it smooth and steady.

6. Repeat the movement for your desired number of repetitions. Show those glutes who's boss!

Some extra tips to keep your hip bridge game strong:

• Control is key! Keep those movements smooth and controlled, avoiding any jerky or wild swings. We want to be the masters of grace and precision.

• Focus on driving through those heels of yours as you lift those hips. Activate those glutes and hamstrings like they're on a mission to save the world.

• Watch that back of yours! Keep it neutral and straight throughout the exercise. No excessive arching or rounding—we're aiming for the perfect posture here.

• Keep that core engaged, just like a fortress protecting your lower back. Stabilize that torso and let those abs do their work.

• Need some extra stability? Plant those palms on the ground, facing down, for an added boost. Or feel free to experiment with different arm positions as you become more confident in your hip bridge mastery.

• Ready to level up? Try out some single-leg hip bridges or add a resistance band above your knees for some extra resistance.

The hip bridge exercise is a fantastic addition to your lower body or full-body workout routine. Embrace that booty power and bridge your way to glorious glutes and a strong lower back.

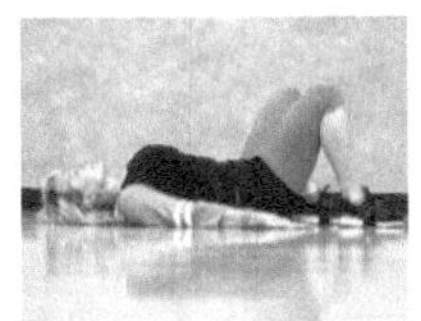 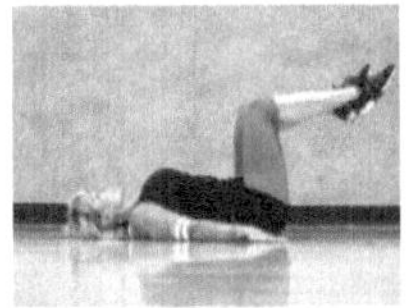 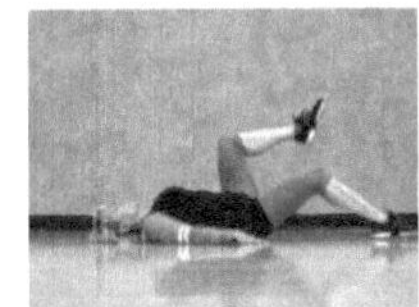

3. SUPINE REVERSE MARCHES:

Alright, let's get marching, but in a reverse kind of way! We're about to target those glutes, hamstrings, and core with some supine reverse marches. Trust me, it's as fun as it sounds! Here's how to do it:

1. Time to lay back and get comfy! Find a squishy exercise mat or a comfy surface to lie on. Bend those knees of yours and plant your feet firmly on the ground, about hip-width apart. Your arms can chill by your sides, palms facing down.
2. Engage that core power! Picture yourself as the captain of a strong and stable ship. Draw your belly button in towards your spine, activating those core muscles and stabilizing your entire torso. You're the captain of stability!
3. Lift both of those fabulous feet off the ground, bringing your knees towards your chest. Now, your thighs should be standing tall, perpendicular to the ground, while your lower legs are chillin' parallel to the ground.
4. Keep that 90-degree angle going strong. Slowly lower your right foot towards the ground while maintaining that hip and knee position.
5. Bring that right foot back up to the starting position while, at the same time, lowering your left foot towards the ground. It's a magical alternating act!
6. Keep the marching rhythm alive! Continue lifting and lowering your legs, as if you're marching like a reverse superstar. Make sure to engage that core and maintain your stability throughout. You're a marching maestro!
7. Repeat the movement for your desired number of repetitions on each leg. March on!

Some extra tips to keep you marching strong:

• Control is key! Keep those movements nice and controlled, avoiding any jerky or wild swinging motions. We're marching with finesse here!

• Embrace those glutes and hamstrings! Focus on using those powerhouse muscles to lift and lower your legs, rather than relying solely on momentum. They're the stars of the show!

• Keep that spine of yours neutral and fabulous throughout the exercise. No arching or rounding allowed—let's keep it strong and stable.

• Keep that core engaged! It's your secret weapon for stability and lower back protection. Brace yourself!

• Ready for some extra challenge? Strap on some ankle weights or resistance bands around those ankles of yours. Let's level up the marching game!

Supine reverse marches are a fantastic addition to your lower body or core workout routine. It's a marching extravaganza that targets those glutes, hamstrings, and core like nothing else. So get ready to march your way to strength and stability. You're the captain of this reverse march parade!

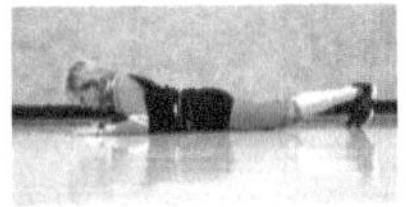 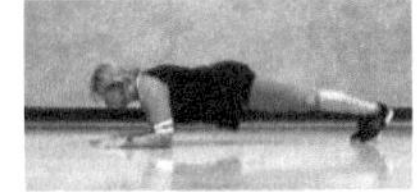

4.PLANK:

Alright, it's time to get down and plank-y! The plank exercise is here to strengthen that core of yours and give those abs, back, and stabilizing muscles a serious workout. Let's dive into the step-by-step guide:

1. Get yourself comfortable! Lay face down on a squishy exercise mat or any cozy surface you can find. Plant your forearms on the ground, making sure your elbows are right under your shoulders. Your arms should be parallel to each other, about shoulder-width apart. We're building a solid foundation here!

2. Extend those legs straight back, resting on your tippy toes. Now, imagine a straight line running from your head all the way down to your heels. Engage that core power by sucking that belly button in towards your spine. We're ready to rock!

3. Keep that neck of yours neutral. Look down at the ground, keeping your head in line with your body. Slowly lift your body off the floor, maintaining a stiff torso and legs. You're like a strong plank, unmovable!

4. Hold this plank position, with your core engaged and body straight as an arrow, for as long as you can handle. We're talking endurance here! Start with shorter durations, like 20 to 30 seconds, and then gradually increase the time as you build up those mighty core muscles.

5. Don't forget to breathe! Inhale and exhale steadily, like a zen master, throughout the exercise. We're all about that controlled breathing here.

6. When it's time to wrap it up, slowly lower your body back down to the floor and relax. You've nailed that plank!

Here are some extra tips to keep you planking like a pro:

• Keep those movements under control No sagging or lifting those hips too high. Your body should be in a straight line from your head to your heels. Think of yourself as a plank—solid and strong!

• Focus on engaging that core of yours throughout the exercise. Your arms and shoulders are just there for support. It's all about that core power!

• No holding your breath! Breathe naturally and continuously, like a gentle breeze, throughout the exercise. Inhale the power, exhale the strength.

• Relax those shoulders and keep them away from your ears. No shrugging or tensing allowed! Keep that neck and shoulders steady throughout the plank.

• If your lower back is feeling a bit uncomfortable, no worries! Modify the exercise by doing a forearm plank with your knees resting on the ground. It's all about finding what works best for you.

• Once you're feeling like a plank master, you can level up the challenge! Increase the duration, try variations like side planks, or even go for some plank leg lifts.

The plank exercise can be a star player in your core workout routine or as part of a full-body workout.

STATIC STRETCHES FOR EACH MAJOR BODY GROUP

Alrighty, let's get those muscles all stretched out and feeling groovy! Here's a bunch of standing stretches for each major body part. No need to lay down or do anything fancy. We're keeping it simple and fun!

1. **Neck:**
    • **Neck Side Stretch**: Tilt your head to the side like you're trying to touch your ear to your shoulder. Hold it there for a cool 20-30 seconds on each side. Feel the stretch!
    • **Neck Rotation Stretch:** Slowly turn your head like you're checking out what's happening behind you. Hold that peek-a-boo position for 20-30 seconds on each side. It's like being a curious owl!
    • **Neck Flexion Stretch:** Drop your chin towards your chest and feel the stretch in the back of your neck. Hold it there for a good 20-30 seconds. Keep your eyes on your toes!
    • **Neck Extension Stretch:** Look up to the sky and gently arch your neck backward. Hold it for 20-30 seconds. Hello, up there!
    • **Neck Lateral Flexion Stretch:** Tilt your head to the side and give it an extra oomph by gently pulling it with your hand. Hold that stretch for 20-30 seconds on each side. Stretch and tug!

2. **Shoulders:**

• **Shoulder Arm Across Stretch**: Extend one arm straight out in front of you and give it a big hug across your chest with your other hand. Hold it tight for 20-30 seconds on each side. Spread the love!

• **Shoulder Behind-the-Back Stretch**: Reach one arm behind your back like you're trying to tickle yourself. Can you touch your other hand? Hold it for 20-30 seconds on each side. That's some back-reaching action!

• **Shoulder Overhead Stretch**: Raise one arm up and over your head, reaching towards the opposite side. Feel that stretch! Hold it for 20-30 seconds on each side. Wave hello to the sky!

• **Shoulder Circle Stretch**: Time to shake those shoulders! Rotate them in big circles, forwards and backwards. Loosen up those muscles and improve your mobility. It's like doing the shoulder dance!

3. **Chest:**

• **Chest Wall Stretch**: Stand facing a wall and put your forearm against it at shoulder height. Now gently twist your body away from the wall and feel that sweet chest stretch. Hold it for 20-30 seconds on each side. Wall, meet chest!

• **Doorway Chest Stretch**: Find a doorway and place your forearms on the door frame. Step forward a bit and feel the stretch in your chest. Hold it for 20-30 seconds. Embrace the door frame!

• **Standing Chest Opener**: Interlace your fingers behind your back, squeeze those shoulder blades together, and lift your arms away from your body. Open up that chest! Hold it for 20-30 seconds.

• **Arm Across Chest Stretch**: Give yourself a cozy hug by bringing one arm across your chest. Use your other hand to pull it closer. Hold it for 20-30 seconds on each side. Hug it out!

• **Chest Expansion Stretch**: Extend both arms behind you and clasp your hands together. Gently lift your arms away from your body and feel that chest stretch. Hold it for 20-30 seconds. Expand and conquer!

4. **Back:**

• **Standing Back Extension Stretch**: Put your hands on your lower back and slowly arch backward, looking up at the ceiling. It's like doing a limbo dance! Hold that arch for 20-30 seconds. Limbo your back!

• **Standing Spinal Twist**: Stand with your feet hip-width apart and twist your torso to one side. Hold onto something stable for support. Feel that twisty goodness! Hold it for 20-30 seconds on each side. Let's twist again!

• **Standing Forward Bend**: Stand with your feet hip-width apart and fold forward from your hips. Let your upper body hang down towards your toes or the floor. It's like being a ragdoll! Hold that chill pose for 20-30 seconds. Hang loose!

• **Standing Side Bend**: Reach one arm overhead and lean to the opposite side. Feel the stretch along your side. Hold it for 20-30 seconds on each side. Side-to-side goodness!

• **Standing Cat-Cow Stretch**: Bend over and round your back like a Halloween cat, and then stay bent over and arch your back. Repeat the movement for a few breaths. Meow and moo! Let the animal inside you shine!

5. **Hamstrings:**

• **Standing Hamstring Stretch**: Stand tall and extend one leg forward with a slight bend in the knee. Hinge forward at the hips and reach towards your toes. It's like saying hi to your foot! Hold it for 20-30 seconds on each leg. Toe touch time!

• **Standing Quad Stretch with Hamstring Emphasis**: Stand tall, lift one foot up behind you, and grab your ankle. Pull your foot towards your glutes while keeping your knee pointing downward. Stretch that quad and hamstring! Hold it for 20-30 seconds on each leg. Get flexible!

• **Standing Wide-Leg Forward Fold**: Stand with your feet wider than shoulder-width apart and reach towards the ground. It's like being a human triangle! Hold that wide-legged fold for 20-30 seconds.

• **Standing Hamstring Stretch with Hip Hinge**: Stand with one foot slightly in front of the other and hinge forward at the hips, reaching towards the ground. It's like you're saying hi to the floor! Hold it for 20-30 seconds on each leg. Say hello to the floor!

6. **Quadriceps:**

• **Standing Quad Stretch with Bent Knee**: Stand tall, grab your ankle, and pull your heel towards your glutes. Keep that knee pointing downward to feel the quad stretch. Hold it for 20-30 seconds on each leg. Quad power!

• **Standing Quad Stretch with Side Reach**: Stand tall, grab your ankle, and pull your heel towards your glutes. Now reach your opposite arm overhead and gently lean to the side. Stretch that quad and side body! Hold it for 20-30 seconds on each leg. Reach and stretch!

• **Standing Quad Stretch with Hip Extension**: Stand tall, grab your ankle, and pull your heel towards your glutes. Push your hip forward slightly to intensify the quad stretch. Hold it for 20-30 seconds on each leg. Show off those quads!

7. **Calves:**

• **Standing Calf Stretch with Wall**: Stand facing a wall, put your hands on the wall at shoulder height, and step one foot back, keeping your back leg straight. Lean forward to stretch your calf. Hold it for 20-30 seconds on each leg. Give that calf a wall high-five!

• **Standing Calf Stretch with Lunge:** Step one foot forward into a lunge position, keeping your back leg straight and your heel flat on the ground. Lean forward to stretch your calf. Hold it for 20-30 seconds on each leg. Lunge and stretch!

• **Standing Calf Stretch with Heel Raise**: Stand with the balls of your feet on the edge of a step or curb. Lower your heels down to stretch your calves, and then raise your heels up for a slight calf raise. Hold that stretch position for 20-30 seconds. Calves on the edge!

8. **Hips:**
   • **Sitting Hip Stretch**: While sitting on a chair, cross your right leg over your left leg and rest it on your left thigh. Feel that hip stretch! Hold it for 20-30 seconds. Then switch to the other leg. Cross and stretch!

Remember to take it easy and enjoy these stretches. No bouncing or jerking allowed! Hold each stretch for 20-30 seconds, or whatever feels comfortable for you. And don't forget to take deep breaths while you stretch—it's like giving your muscles a little vacation. Stretching is all about finding your sweet spot and having a blast while taking care of your body. So, let's get stretching and have some fun!

TEN THINGS TO ALWAYS REMEMBER

Hey there, senior superstar! It's time to dive into the world of fitness and have a blast while taking care of your amazing self. Here are ten key points to keep in mind as you embark on this adventure:

1. **Consult your doctor**: Before you become the fitness guru that you are, have a chat with your doc to make sure everything's in tip-top shape. They'll give you the green light and provide any helpful advice for your unique situation. Doctor's orders!

2. **Start slow**: Rome wasn't built in a day, and neither will your fitness empire. Begin with exercises that make your heart sing, but at a low intensity. Then, as you get comfortable, gradually crank up the heat. Remember, slow and steady wins the race!

3. **Warm up and cool down**: It's like giving your body a warm hug before and after your workouts. Start with light cardio to get your blood pumping, and do some dynamic stretches to limber up those muscles. After your sweat session, cool down with some gentle moves to help your body recover. You've got this!

4. **Focus on proper form**: Think of yourself as a fitness Picasso—every move you make is a work of art. Pay attention to your technique and make sure you're doing each exercise correctly. It's like sculpting your muscles while keeping injuries at bay. You're a form master!

5. **Listen to your body**: Your body is a smart cookie, so tune in to its messages. If something doesn't feel right or you're pushing your limits too hard, take a breather. You're not a superhero (well, maybe you

are!), so give yourself permission to rest and seek professional advice if needed. You're the boss of your body!

6. **Mix it up**: Variety is the spice of life! Keep things exciting by trying different exercises. Go for a walk one day, lift some weights the next, and maybe throw in some balance exercises and flexibility work too. Your body will thank you, and you'll never get bored. Keep it spicy!

7. **Hydrate adequately**: Water, water everywhere! Stay hydrated by sipping on that good ol' H2O before, during, and after your workouts. It's like giving your body a refreshing waterfall. Dehydration is no fun, so keep that water bottle by your side. Stay quenched!

8. **Use appropriate equipment**: Time to gear up like a fitness pro! Make sure you have comfy shoes and any necessary supportive equipment for your exercises. Safety first!

9. **Rest and recover**: You're a fitness warrior, but even warriors need to recharge their batteries. Give your body some downtime to rest and recover between workouts. It's like pressing the pause button on your workout playlist. Rest and be your awesome self!

10. **Have realistic goals**: It's time to dream big, but keep it real too. Set goals that you can achieve and track your progress along the way. SMART goals are the name of the game—Specific, Measurable, Attainable, Relevant, and Time-bound. You're a goal-getting superstar!

Remember, you're unique, so tailor your program to fit your needs. Don't hesitate to seek guidance from fitness pros like personal trainers or physical therapists—they're like your personal fitness cheerleaders. Let's rock this fitness journey, senior style!